The New Yoga for Healthy Aging

Living Longer, Living Stronger, and Loving Every Day

Suza Francina

Photographs by Jim Jacobs

Health Communications, Inc.
Deerfield Beach, Florida

www.bcibooks.com

Before beginning any exercise program, please consult with your physician.

Library of Congress Cataloging-in-Publication Data

Francina, Suza.

The new yoga for healthy aging : living longer, living stronger and loving
    every day / Suza Francina ; photographs by Jim Jacobs.
        p. cm.
    Includes bibliographical references and index.
    ISBN-13: 978-0-7573-0532-0 (trade paper)
    ISBN-10: 0-7573-0532-6 (trade paper)
1. Yoga—Health aspects.   2. Aging—Prevention.   I. Title.
    RA781.7.F68 2007
    613.7′046—dc22

                                                                    2006039372

©2007 Suza Francina

Publisher: Health Communications, Inc.
                3201 S.W. 15th Street
                Deerfield Beach, FL 33442-8190

Photos of Bernard Spira by Garth McLean
Photo of Eleanor Williams by Jodi Robbins
Cover and inside photos ©Jim Jacobs
Cover design by Andrea Perrine Brower
Interior book design by Lawna Patterson Oldfield

Praise for *The New Yoga for Healthy Aging*

"*The New Yoga for Healthy Aging* is one of the most exciting yoga books ever published. Its promise is one that millions of baby boomers will find comforting—that yoga is a natural prescription for reversing the aging process. The proof is in the lovely and inspiring photographs of yoga students in their later years in poses of beauty and strength. This outstanding resource addresses the common ailments of aging and is as encouraging as it is informative and practical. Suza Francina shows how even challenging yoga poses become 'do-able' through the use of props and modifications. Her extensive knowledge and experience teaching yoga is evident, and her wisdom and deep caring shine through her words and stories."

—Peggy Cappy
Author, *Yoga for All of Us,* and creator of the popular video series
Yoga for the Rest of Us, as seen on public television, and the audio CD
series *Deep Relaxation for the Rest of Your Life*

"What a delight to read of 'seniors' who are choosing to live life to the fullest and touching their toes while they do it! I felt inspired and hopeful when I read this book, not only for our world, but also for myself as I age. In fact, I think I will step on my yoga mat right now and enjoy the fruits of Suza's long experience and clear suggestions. I feel younger already! I strongly recommend this book for all levels of practitioners as well as for yoga teachers."

—Judith Hanson Lasater, Ph.D., P.T.
Yoga teacher since 1971, and author of
six books, including *A Year of Living Your Yoga*

"Suza Francina's book is an essential guide for yoga teachers to meet the challenge of the huge wave of people moving into their sixties and seventies. We need to show capable older men and women that they don't have to limit themselves to the simplest poses! Suza's book is for everyone who wants to grow old with grace and strength beyond what they ever imagined possible!"

—Maggie Spilner
Author of *Walk Your Way Through Menopause*

"I currently teach yoga in a wellness center for seniors under the auspices of California State University and highly recommend all of Suza's books to my students as well as to other yoga teachers. Suza's books emphasize and celebrate the beauty and wisdom of the older practitioner. At sixty years of age, I never cease to be inspired and energized by the stories and pictures of my fellow yogis featured in her books and by Suza's obvious deep regard for older adults and her love of yoga. Suza has found a way to put a 'face' (and a smiling one at that) on yoga for older adults. Her books are more than 'how-to-do manuals' on yoga—they explain 'why we should' do yoga which is why I love to share them. I consider them yoga book gems!"

—Janice Freeman-Bell, R.Y.T.
California State University and Sierra Center for Yoga Studies

"Suza Francina is an extraordinary yoga teacher, deeply knowledgeable of the field and so skilled in passing on the joy of yoga. Her new book leads students safely and comfortably through a wide variety of poses. She knows the idiosyncrasies of the older population and describes appropriate props and pose variations to be used when needed. We are privileged to have Suza's expert guidance available in this book!"

—Judith Vander
Seventy-year-old yoga student

"Suza Francina presents yoga in a way that that creates confidence in readers to be independent and strong."

—B. K. S. Iyengar
From the Foreword of *The New Yoga for People Over 50*

To Malchia Olshan

*Who always reminded us that
if we can't laugh at ourselves when we
wake up in the morning, we
shouldn't get out of bed.*

———————

*"Start your morning with yoga,
wear beads while baking,
make brownies and enjoy life!!"*

—MALCHIA OLSHAN

CONTENTS

ACKNOWLEDGMENTS

Writing a book is a long voyage, and many friendly souls have accompanied me along the way.

It all begins with a good agent, and Barbara Neighbors Deal is the best. She held my hand from long distance through all the difficult passages and reminded me: "Take a deep breath and let it be easy."

Jim Jacobs, the photographer for this book, is a consummate professional. With the assistance of his son, Alex Jacobs Hirth, he produced the images that grace and enliven the pages of this book.

My appreciation to all the models who gave so generously of their time and yoga expertise: Ramanand Patel, Betty Eiler, Barbara Wiechmann, Judith Alper, Lewis Perry, Olney Fortier, Tsuneko Hellerstein, Lillian Cartwright, Neti Fredericks, Margaret Ghuman, Parminder Singh Ghuman, Josefina Vigne, Karen Breslin, Judy Goldhalft, Eleanor Williams, Bernard Spira, Nora Burnett, and Toni Montez.

Thanks also to the Berkeley Yoga Center and Bija Yoga in San Francisco for the use of their beautiful yoga studio space.

I want to thank all the contributors whose stories illuminate the themes of this book. There are many others whose friendship, assistance, and ideas energized me "behind the scenes" to complete this project: Shirley Shapiro, David Shapiro, Susan Winter Ward, Jane Fryer, Lolly Font, and Maggie Spilner.

David E. Moody, Ph.D., is my West Coast editor and collaborator. Like the shoemaker's elves, he took my unrestrained prose at the end of the day and tamed it overnight. He often reminded me that I wasn't writing the encyclopedia of yoga. If not for him, by now I might be on page 1,000 of chapter 1!

Thank you, Susan Clark, for typing, proofreading, and contributing editorial services so that I could take a yoga nap.

Carin Seebold provided expert editorial advice from the point of view of a yoga student.

Diana Kelly's eagle eyes and magical file transmission abilities kept the manuscript machinery well-oiled and in motion.

Special thanks to everyone at Health Communications, Inc.—Peter Vegso, president of HCI; Allison Janse and Carol Rosenberg, who guided the book through the editorial process; Andrea Perrine Brower for her cover design; Lawna Patterson Oldfield for the text layout and design; Larissa Hise Henoch; and Kim Weiss and the rest of the talented HCI staff.

My intrepid copyeditor was Heath Lynn Silberfeld in southern Florida. Publishing a book without any mistakes is nearly impossible, but she overcame all obstacles, including the author, to make that happen.

A student never forgets the teacher who initiates her into the practice of yoga. Only now that I am almost as old as my first instructor, Sarah Kirton, have I come to fully appreciate how she invited me into her living room to join her yoga group. She waived the four-dollar tuition so that I could hire a babysitter. When she moved away in 1972, I inherited her classes at a senior center, and that's how I discovered my calling.

The seeds for my books for people at midlife and older were nurtured by many other teachers, most especially Felicity Green, Beverly Graves, Toni Montez, Mary Dunn, Judith Hanson Lasater, Patricia Sullivan, and Elise Miller.

The highlight of many of my writing days occurred when my ten-year-old niece, Olivia Klein, would quietly open the door, peek inside, and ask, "Have you eaten?" And then she would deliver something delicious, prepared by my sister, Paula Klein.

I am very grateful too for the love and support of my parents, Mary and Rene Diets, my sister Maria, and my children, Bo and Monica.

Virginia Lee gave me nurturing energy and heavenly massages to get the kinks out of my shoulders after a long day at the keyboard. My friends Dale Hanson, Debbie Watson, Peggy La Cerra, and Christine Golden made me forget deadlines and feel carefree again!

Above all, I can never fully repay Sholom Joshua for his editing, proofreading, love, and support—and for taking Trixie, Beau, and Queenie on long walks and keeping the cupboard well-stocked with Fancy Feast for Tiny Cat.

With their wonderfully flexible spines, cats are the yoga masters of the animal world—even while they lounge on the keyboard and my papers. My days are enriched by their presence: Princess Priscilla, the model child; her bullying brother, Leo the Lion; solitary, cross-eyed Ginger Cat; the orphan interloper, Spot; and contemplative, congenial Pierre.

Last but certainly not least, my thanks in memoriam to The Great Being, Rosie the pot-bellied pig.

FOREWORD

The ancient practice of Hatha yoga views a healthy body as a sanctuary for spiritual awakening. This more than two-thousand-year-old discipline was integrated into a broader social vision of "stages of life," where each individual moved from earlier stages more engaged in the material world—such as having a job and raising a family—to later stages that encouraged separation from material responsibilities to pursue enlightenment.

In approaching aging in the modern world, Suza Francina returns to this ancient perspective of the later stages of life, not as something to be endured or suffered through, but as a celebration and opportunity to reach deeper into ourselves—growing in wisdom, compassion, and joy. In this comprehensive, informative, and engaging book, she convincingly demonstrates that yoga practice can prompt both spiritual and physical transformation, helping people safely gain and maintain strength and flexibility—and reduce pain and suffering—with age.

Yoga is an ideal form of movement for older adults for many reasons. Under the guidance of a well-qualified instructor, yoga involves non-competitive, mindful movement that encourages people to start where they are, breathe deeply, and release tension. Today's seniors have a broad range of abilities—from being unable to climb a single stair to running triathlons—and yoga offers a unique means of optimizing health at an individual level. For someone in a wheelchair or hospital bed, yoga practice might simply be learning how to take a deep abdominal breath. Another senior's practice might involve discovering how to stand securely on two feet or to balance on just one. And for strong, agile elders, such as the inspiring yogis and yoginis pictured in this book, yoga offers a limitless opportunity to "grow young" by engaging in the myriad joys of move-ment—twisting, bending, and even turning the world upside down.

Another benefit for aging bodies is that—unlike the Western "no pain, no gain" mindset—yoga involves chal-lenge *without strain*. As the sage Patanjali wrote in the classic text on yoga, the *Yoga Sutras*, a posture should have the dual qualities of *alertness* and *relaxation*—or, as the text is some-times translated, *steadiness* and *comfort*. Forcing and over-exertion—with the accompanying risk of injury—has no place in yoga practice.

But even more important than yoga's physical benefits are the mental, emotional, and spiritual aspects of the practice. Yoga is much more than just exercise, it is a form of holistic self-care designed to enhance energy and boost wellness. Since disease is considered an obstacle to enlightenment, ancient yogis designed these practices to help people become healthy and strong enough to bring the mind into stillness and connect with the divine. This makes yoga a particularly potent practice for those facing their own physical limitations and mortality itself.

In recent years, modern science has confirmed this ancient yogic understanding of the healing power of movement. This is particularly important in our aging society since a growing body of evidence suggests that regular, moderate exercise—such as yoga—is as close as we may come to a true fountain of youth. Study after study shows that physical activity can prevent, relieve—and sometimes even cure—a host of ailments that often accompany aging. These ailments will reach epidemic proportions as the wave of "baby boomers" advance into and beyond their sixth decade of life, and many will survive for an additional two decades or more.

Regular exercise can help some diabetics come off insulin and some hypertensives quit their high blood-pressure medication. It can lower cholesterol, ease arthritis pain, lift depression, relieve anxiety, and help asthmatics breathe more easily. Appropriate activity can strengthen muscles and preserve bone, even in the frail elderly, allowing some in their eighties and nineties to double and triple their strength to the point where many are able to walk and perform other tasks without assistance. At a time when nursing homes are filled with seniors who are institutionalized—not because of disease or cognitive impairment, but because their muscles are so weak that they need help with simple tasks, like getting up out of a chair—physical activity such as yoga holds great promise as a low-cost, low-risk, effective way to retain independence with age.

In fact, the healing power of movement is so strong that a

report from the National Institute on Aging states: "If exercise could be packed into a pill, it would be the single most widely prescribed, and beneficial medicine in the nation."

As one of America's pioneers in the growing field of teaching yoga to seniors, Suza Francina is uniquely qualified to guide older adults and their teachers in the art and science of yoga practice for healthy aging. This book distills her more than thirty years of experience in teaching, and being taught by, older adults, and the resulting resource is remarkable—both as a practical, how-to manual as well as a moving tribute to yoga's potential for transformation at any age.

Carol first "met" Suza by telephone in 1998, when she interviewed her for a Bodyworks column, which ran in the *Washington Post* on April 28 under the headline: "Standing the Aging Process on Its Head: For Some Seniors, Yoga Is a Fountain of Strength and Flexibility." In the article, Suza recalled how she first discovered the rejuvenating effects of yoga in the early 1970s, when she began studying yoga with a sixty-five-year-old neighbor and several older teachers, including an eighty-four-year-old man. Then in her twenties, Suza had been working with seniors since age fourteen, when she began assisting elderly neighbors in her Ojai, California, community—befriending and caring for many of them until they died. The difference between the seniors who taught her yoga and those she assisted was stunning.

"Here were these vital people with beautiful posture, who were the same age as some of the frail people I took care of," she said. "The contrast was striking. It made me realize that we live in a chair-and-car culture, and the cold reality is that people who don't use their legs lose them." When one of her teachers moved away, Suza took over teaching her yoga class at a retirement home and discovered that, over time, even students in their eighties and nineties could grow stronger and more flexible. "As a teacher," she said. "I find it a continual revelation to see how the bodies of people of all ages respond to yoga and proper exercise."

Suza challenged the then-conventional wisdom that aging is a process of stiffening, rigidity, and closing down and recognized that much of the disability associated with age actually comes from disuse. Yoga postures move "each joint in the body through its full range of motion—stretching, strengthening and balancing each part," said Suza, who began sharing these insights in 1977, with her first book, *Yoga for People Over 50.* She continued to offer advice and encouragement in ensuing volumes, *The New Yoga for People Over 50* in 1997 and *Yoga and the Wisdom of Menopause* in 2003.

With this latest book, Suza continues to counter negative stereotypes of aging with remarkable photographs of seemingly ageless yogis and yoginis and truly touching stories of yoga's deep impact on older adult's bodies, minds, and spirits. She offers insights into dealing with the most common health challenges facing older adults—including osteoporosis, arthritis, hip replacement, hypertension, and Parkinson's disease. Suza approaches her subject and her students with respect and dignity, never talking down or patronizing. Instructions are carefully outlined and safe, but not limiting. The focus throughout is on living each moment as fully and joyfully as possible, regardless of age or health status. *The New Yoga for Healthy Aging* provides a great service in awakening people to what Suza calls "yoga's ascending path to physical and spiritual transformation."

—**Carol Krucoff, R.Y.T.**
Yoga Instructor/Therapist and Journalist

—**Mitchell Krucoff, M.D.**
Professor of Medicine/Cardiology,
Duke University Medical Center

Authors of *Healing Moves: How to Cure, Relieve, and Prevent Common Ailments with Exercise* (www.healingmoves.com)

INTRODUCTION

*Yoga brings gifts from your very first day.
These benefits can be experienced even by raw beginners,
who feel something beginning to happen at a deep level in
their bodies, in their minds, and even in their souls.
Some describe the first gifts as a new feeling of lightness or
calm or joy. The miracle is that after seventy years, these
gifts are still increasing for me. . . . If you think that
learning to touch your toes or even stand on your head is
the whole of yoga, you have missed most of its bounty,
most of its blessings, and most of its beauty.*

B. K. S. Iyengar, *Light on Life*

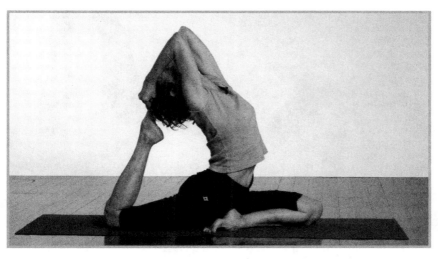

**Barbara Wiechmann, age 63, demonstrates One-Legged King Pigeon Pose,
Eka Pada Rajakapotasana I.**

Welcome to
The New Yoga for Healthy Aging!

Thirty years have passed since I wrote my first book on yoga for people at midlife and older. In 1977, when I was searching for a publisher for *Yoga for People Over Fifty*, one publisher wondered if the world really needed another yoga book, since there were already so many titles—at least twenty—in print!

At that time, few people imagined that by the turn of the century an explosion of publications would appear on every

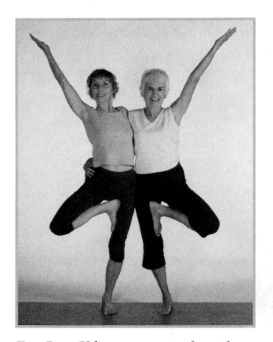

Tree Pose, **Vrksasana,** *strengthens the feet and legs and develops balance and steadiness. Practicing with a partner is fun and helps you stay in the pose longer.*

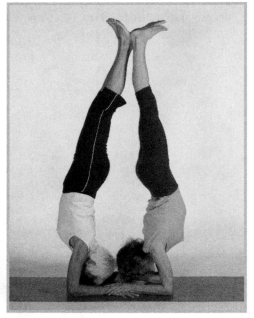

Forearm Balance, Peacock Feather Pose, **Pincha Mayurasana.** *Betty Eiler and Barbara Wiechmann have been practicing together for many years.*

aspect of yoga—from its philosophical and spiritual roots to the integration of yoga and medical science—over 4,000 titles and still growing. When I helped launch a struggling alternative magazine, *Yoga Journal,* I did not dream that yoga would spread like wildfire and that B. K. S. Iyengar, then the virtually unknown author of *Light On Yoga,* would someday be named by *Time* magazine as one of the "100 Most Influential People in the World."

When I see photographs of B. K. S. Iyengar now, at age eighty-eight, demonstrating how he stays for long periods of time in backbends and inverted poses, I realize I am looking at a master role model: a timeless, ageless practitioner who is showing the world what healthy aging really looks like.

In this book you will meet a wide range of inspiring role models, many who began yoga in their fifties, sixties, seventies, and older. Others are longtime teachers, such as Shirley Daventry French, in her mid-seventies, who says, "I'm not *getting* old. I *am* old!" Thank goodness these modern-day yogis are not recluses living in mountaintop caves, and that they are here and willing to share their wisdom, insights, challenges, and successes with us!

As seventy-year-old yoga teacher Eleanor Williams points out, "There is a vast difference between young old age and *old* old age!" Even if you are someone who considers sixty as "the new forty," the issues we face in our sixties have a heightened intensity. The challenges at this stage of life—and how we choose to approach them—will determine to a great extent the quality of our later years.

*Those of us who have the privilege of
being a part of this historical new collaboration
of Western medicine and yoga are witness to
a beautiful new friendship that will continue
to reform the face of healthcare in the
twenty-first century and beyond.*

Nirmala Heriza, author of *Dr. Yoga* and a Hatha yoga
cardiac therapist, Cedars-Sinai Medical Center
Preventive and Rehabilitative Cardiac Center

Yoga Solutions for Healthy Aging

It is a fact that as we age the human body has a natural tendency to become increasingly rigid and inflexible. The body of the young child is exceptionally pliable. Even as young adults, we still retain the capacity to move and bend in every direction. The loss of this capacity is a defining hallmark of old age.

Of all the forms and systems of exercise devised by human beings, yoga is preeminent in its ability to preserve and extend our youthful suppleness. Indeed, there is no other science or system of activity that even attempts, as yoga does, to comprehensively address this particular aspect of physical function. To be sure, yoga has many other fundamental benefits, but the attention to flexibility is among its foremost gifts.

For this reason alone, yoga is the most natural and essential remedy for the effects of aging. If reason ruled the world, most yoga classes would be populated disproportionately by the middle-aged and older! Yoga is their natural ally. Instead, most

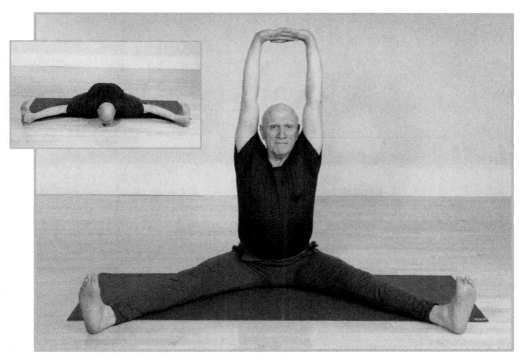

Seated Wide-Angle Pose, **Upavistha Konasana,** *keeps the spine, hip joints, and thigh muscles flexible.*

yoga classes consist primarily of students in their twenties, thirties, and forties. As good as yoga is for those age groups, it is even more important as we get older. The fundamental aim of this book is to convey that message in all of its many and varied applications.

Even though yoga has entered the fitness mainstream, its full potential as a preventive and rehabilitative component in holistic, cutting-edge gerontology is just beginning to be explored. In the last ten years, research has documented the effectiveness of yoga for improving many health conditions. As 78 million baby boomers (one in every five Americans) move

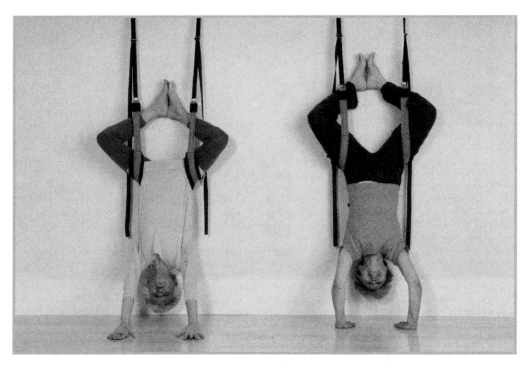

Hanging upside down in a pelvic sling allows people of all ages to reap the rejuvenating benefits of Headstand, **Sirsasana,** *without straining the neck.*

into the time of life when chronic conditions combine with the long-term wear and tear on their bodies, more and more of them will turn to yoga for both prevention and rehabilitation.

In *The New Yoga for Healthy Aging,* you will learn about the integration of yoga and Western medicine and what the emerging fields of yoga therapy and holistic gerontology have to offer for building a foundation for healthy aging. You will meet "Yoga doctors," such as Krishna Raman, M.D., Timothy McCall, M.D., and others, whose writings on therapeutic yoga are invaluable resources for yoga teachers, medical doctors, and other health practitioners.

Even though yoga is now mainstream, the sight of an elderly person hanging upside down from a pelvic sling, lying over a Backbender, or practicing standing poses with the support of a "horse" is still unusual. Our society recognizes the need for products that help older people maintain their independence: mobility aids such as canes, walkers, transport chairs, and scooters and safety devices such as grab bars, shower benches, and nonskid mats. We don't consider such things luxuries, but rather necessities. In the coming years, I believe we will see a paradigm shift in which yoga props will be viewed in a similar way.

When I began learning yoga, I was also working as a home healthcare provider for frail elders, some confined to a wheelchair and bed. I cared for many of the same people into the last years of their lives, often helping them through the dying process. I had the opportunity to observe firsthand the mental and physical changes that commonly occur in the later years. I saw how life can change in an instant after a stroke and how the body can linger for many years, long after the mind is gone.

People sometimes tell me, "But not everyone can afford to go to a yoga class or purchase those expensive yoga bolsters." One reader even accused me of being "elitist," arguing that many older people cannot afford to attend classes at fully equipped yoga centers and that they don't have the money to purchase props for home use.

My reply is this: one year of yoga costs less than a single day in the hospital. This book gives convenient alternatives to standard props for situations in which they are truly not available, but I urge you to think of the yoga props shown throughout this book as preventive medicine. The National Academy of

Sciences has reported that if the average age of institutionalization could be postponed by just one month, it would save over
$3 billion in Medicare and Medicaid—and that figure doesn't
encompass the priceless savings in dignity and independence
for elderly people.

I believe that someday yoga chairs, bolsters, wall ropes,
pelvic slings, and even Backbenders will seem as normal as
any other common item. In the coming years, more doctors
will follow the lead of today's mind–body medicine pioneers
and will have props and yoga therapy programs available in
medical offices, hospitals, and senior wellness centers.
Insurance companies and Medicare are acknowledging that
programs promoting health and balance, and preventing falls
and other accidents, deserve coverage.

A Word About Yoga Books

No single book, not even one the size of a large reference work,
can possibly tell you all there is to know about yoga. I have a col-
lection of over a hundred yoga books, including the first book by
Indra Devi, published in 1960, and an autographed first edition
of B. K. S. Iyengar's classic *Light on Yoga*. My library includes all
the books on teaching yoga to older people. If it has "forever
young," "young at heart," "fountain of youth," "senior," "ageless,"
"agile at 80," or "easy does it" in the title, I probably have it.

These books tell the story of the evolution and adaptation of
yoga in modern Western culture and of the changing view of
aging. The authors of these books were all pioneers, who have
boldly proclaimed that people over fifty are not over the hill

and have championed the concept of yoga and healthy aging way ahead of its time.

How This Book Is Organized

In many ways, writing a book on yoga is like teaching a mixed-level yoga course. In the present case, the course is mainly for people at midlife and older, but younger people are welcome to attend! In every class I teach, I look at the people before me to see what they need.

As in a real-life class, the readers of this book represent a wide range of totally unique people. Many of the more experienced students attend class regularly and are eager to practice and learn more. Other students are new or attend class sporadically. Some are unsteady on their feet and unsure about getting down to and back up from the floor. Any of these students may be coming to yoga class to help cope with a broad range of health issues. Also among the readers of this book are teachers of all ages who come to deepen their own practices and to expand their understanding of older students.

This book is written with the needs of these different readers in mind. The opening chapter gives an overview of the paradigm shift in the healthcare field, which is moving away from focusing on chronic disease toward teaching preventive lifestyle changes. Yoga is an integral part of this change. Chapter 1 also provides a peek into one of my yoga classes, as I know that many newcomers like to observe before they join in!

Beginners learn and are motivated by seeing someone close to their age who is more experienced with yoga. Thus, every chapter is followed by an inspiring story, starting with a photo essay of the two main models for this book, Betty Eiler and Barbara Wiechmann.

Chapters 2, 3, and 4 focus on the special benefits of yoga props in the later years. You will see people ages sixty to over ninety practicing yoga with the help of such household objects as chairs and blankets, as well as special props such as Backbenders and wall ropes. You will learn how to use props to relax and replenish your vital energy reserves and how to slow down the aging process by turning yourself safely upside down.

Chapters 5 through 8 focus on the most common health challenges for the later years: keeping our cardiovascular and skeletal systems healthy; relieving arthritic joints; and using yoga for rehabilitation after hip replacement surgery.

Chapter 9 discusses yoga for neurological conditions such as Parkinson's disease. Chapter 10 is about teaching yoga to seniors. The tips for teaching older students (including how to get down to and back up from the floor) will also help beginners practicing at home.

Chapter 11 presents yoga sequences for healthy aging. You will learn how to organize the poses in this book so that you get the most benefit from your at-home practice. Teachers can also use these sequences of poses to help plan safe and enjoyable classes for older beginners.

Every yoga class ends with *Savasana*, the pose of deep relaxation, also known as Corpse Pose, and Chapter 12 explores this *asana*. We all have to face death. In this chapter, we explore the possibility that yoga can help us prepare for that mysterious transition from the known to the unknown.

The appendices include an extensive bibliography of references and a section with contact information for the teachers, doctors, and organizations mentioned in this book.

A Word About Safety and Common Sense

A qualified teacher knows how to adjust and adapt yoga to students' individual needs and abilities. I want to make it crystal clear that the more advanced postures, all portrayed in the photos in this book by people well over sixty, should be learned only under the guidance of an experienced instructor. Since injuries and accidents can happen more easily to older students, it is even more important to study with teachers who have trained in alignment-based methods of yoga and understand the needs of older people.

Yoga teachers vary widely in training and experience, so choose yours as carefully as you would any other healthcare professional. A comprehensive teacher-training program not only gives information on how to do a pose, but also how to teach the pose to a wide range of people with different needs.

If you are starting yoga and have an existing medical condition, look for a teacher who is willing to consult with your doctor or with another healthcare professional who is knowledgeable about your condition. For example, if you have recently had heart surgery or a hip replacement, it is important for your teacher to have as much information about your specific condition as is available.

The gravitational force of Earth is among the most powerful physical influences on human health. Reversing the

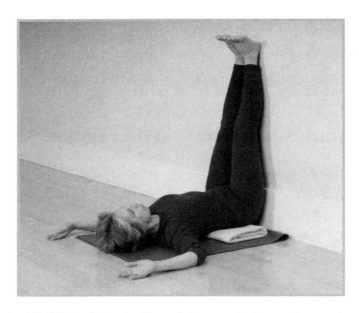

Legs Up the Wall Pose, **Viparita Karani,** *is a gentle inverted pose that removes fatigue from the body.*

gravitational pull by practicing inverted poses is one of the most effective ways of slowing the aging process. Many older people avoid upside-down poses due to their fear of injury. With this book and the right teacher, you can learn how to keep your neck and back healthy and how even octogenarians new to yoga can practice inverted poses safely.

I also want to caution readers not to strain their knees by attempting to sit prematurely in Lotus and related bent-knee postures. Many overly enthusiastic practitioners have learned the hard way that forcing the legs into Lotus can result in serious injury. The practice guidelines in this book will teach you how to safely open your hips without injuring your knees.

The instructions in this book are based on the teachings of B. K. S. Iyengar and his children, Geeta and Prashant Iyengar, all internationally respected authorities on yoga. Standing poses, unique to the Iyengar yoga system, safely strengthen the whole body and are known to relieve many problems related to the aging process. Late-life yoga students with balance problems may *initially* benefit by practicing modified yoga postures while sitting in a chair (see Chapter 3), but practicing in this way can be counterproductive to the goal of keeping older students independent and out of a wheelchair. During my thirty years of teaching yoga to older students, I've learned that most can practice the vital weight-bearing standing poses with the appropriate support of yoga props.

Yoga philosophy teaches that the years after midlife are an ideal time for psychological and spiritual growth. I've written this book for those who reject the notion that aging is an inevitable process of decline and who wish to explore yoga's ascending path to physical and spiritual transformation.

No book can ever replace a yoga teacher who directs, encourages, and inspires you. It is my dream that this book will motivate many more older people to attend yoga classes, thereby increasing their well-being and leading them on the path to healthy aging.

*Namasté,**
Suza Francina
Ojai, California

---

* Namaste *is a traditional expression of greeting and farewell practiced among yogis.* Nama *means "bow,"* as *means "I," and* te *means "you." Therefore,* Namaste *literally means "I bow to you." Its essential meaning is "The divine in me recognizes and honors the divine in you."*

CHAPTER 1

Yoga at Midlife and Beyond: A Journey of Discovery

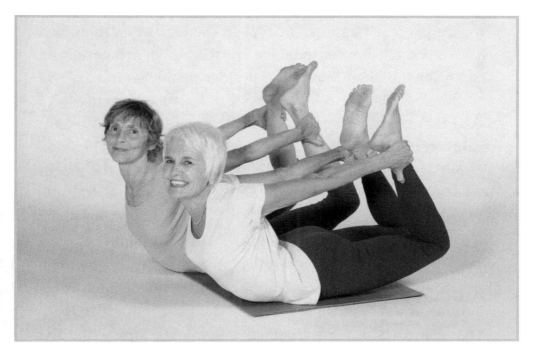

Barbara Wiechmann and Betty Eiler enjoy practicing the Bow Pose. This pose strengthens all the muscles of the back and thus contributes to a youthful, open posture.

Yoga is rightly considered an art. . . .
At the same time, Yoga is also a science. It is
based on ancient observations, principles, and theories
of the mind-body connection, many of which are
now being discovered in medical research.

Larry Payne, Ph.D., cofounder, International
Association of Yoga Therapists and coauthor of *Yoga Rx*

I began teaching yoga in 1972 in the recreation room of a senior citizen center. Like most young, inexperienced teachers, I had the idea that older people were very stiff and fragile and that they might fall or fracture something if I asked them to bend or to balance. I played it safe and taught mainly gentle stretches practiced sitting or lying on the floor. When people told me they had difficulty getting to the floor, I was quick to assure them they could follow the class sitting in a chair.

My perspective on the capacities of older students began to change when I started studying at the Institute for Yoga Teacher Education in San Francisco (now the Iyengar Yoga Institute of San Francisco). There I had the opportunity to observe and assist more seasoned teachers working with their older students. My teachers there revolutionized my views of aging. They took students more than twice my age (then twenty-six) safely, incrementally, into advanced poses such as Full Arm Balance and Upside-Down Bow Pose, which I myself was just beginning to practice.

As I gained experience, I saw that people fifty, sixty, and even older come to yoga with various levels of ability and a wide range of health issues. In over thirty years of teaching, I've learned that most can benefit from the same vital, rejuvenating poses that are taught in my regular classes: standing, inverted, backbending, forward bending, twisting, lying down, and restorative. Now I myself am almost sixty, and my appreciation for the benefits that these poses give in midlife and later years has increased tenfold.

Ancient Yoga Meets Modern Medicine

Yoga's acceptance into the healthcare field is part of a paradigm shift from focusing on chronic disease to focusing on prevention. When cardiologist Dr. Dean Ornish began conducting research thirty years ago on yoga's health benefits, he had to refer to yoga as "stress management techniques" to make it palatable for his patients and colleagues. Dr. Ornish introduced millions to yoga through his studies, published in *Dr. Dean Ornish's Program for Reversing Heart Disease*, showing that heart disease can be reversed through diet, meditation, group support, and yoga. Dr. Ornish now writes a health column for *Newsweek*.

Medicare and other insurance providers will now pay for the cardiac rehabilitation programs created by Dr. Ornish and another mind–body medicine pioneer, Dr. Herbert Benson. Both these doctors have conducted extensive clinical research demonstrating that lifestyle changes—including yoga, meditation, deep breathing and yoga-based relaxation techniques—

may begin to reverse even severe coronary heart disease without drugs or surgery. Drs. Ornish and Benson and their colleagues are also studying the effect of lifestyle intervention programs on other diseases.

Western science is starting to provide concrete data about how yoga works to improve health, prevent disease, and help us cope with and recover from various aches, pains, and illnesses. Research is documenting the effectiveness of yoga therapy and suggesting specific mechanisms for how it works. With increasing precision, scientists are able to look at the brain and body and detect the sometimes subtle changes that practitioners of yoga and meditation undergo.

Timothy McCall, M.D., is another medical doctor whose personal experience with yoga has inspired him to pore over the scientific studies conducted in India and the West to explain how yoga can both prevent disease and help us recover from it. Dr. McCall is a board-certified internist, medical editor for *Yoga Journal,* and author of *Yoga as Medicine.* His website, www.DrMcCall.com, provides a wealth of information on yoga and health.

In the last several decades, those of us in the holistic health field have witnessed an exciting new collaboration between Eastern philosophies of health and Western medicine. A leading Indian physician, Krishna Raman, M.D., has written an encyclopedic book entitled *A Matter of Health: Integration of Yoga and Western Medicine for Prevention and Cure,* which details the physiological effects of yoga poses and the integration of Western medicine with yoga in treating medical disorders. Dr. Raman's book discusses yoga as a medical system that can be applied in the management of a wide range of common ailments. His specialty is the use of yoga props for those who are weak, elderly, or unable to practice postures independently due to illness or accidents. Dr. Raman's ultrasound studies, described in his book *Yoga and Medical Science,* clearly show the exact changes occurring in the blood vessels during the practice of yoga postures.

It is becoming increasingly common for a physician or other primary healthcare provider to recommend a prescription that includes practicing yoga. In 1998 the UCLA School of Medicine became the first U.S. medical school to include a course in yoga (taught by Dr. Larry Payne, coauthor of *Yoga Rx*). Medical schools nationwide are now teaching yoga, and other universities provide yoga education in their medical health departments. Yoga teachers are working with people in hospitals, physical therapy clinics, doctor's offices, and various other types of medical settings. In addition, yoga teachers and doctors are working together to conduct studies on all areas of yoga and health, including the benefits of yoga for an aging population.

You will hear more from the yoga doctors in upcoming chapters. Now let's take a breather and visit one of my yoga classes.

A Peek into My Yoga Class for People at Midlife and Older

It's Monday morning and I'm observing the students warming up in my "Over Fifty" class.

Barbara, age ninety-two, is practicing Half-Moon Pose with her back against the wall, her hand on the seat of a chair. It is empowering for Barbara to practice the same vital weight-bearing poses that younger students practice.

Bob is a sixty-four-year-old man, a newcomer with typically tight hamstrings. He is lying on the floor and stretching his legs with a strap around his foot. I have explained to him that the exercises he has been doing for sixteen years are not removing the stiffness that is settling into his body as he ages. His upper back is rounded from years of desk work, and I place a folded blanket under his head to keep it level while he stretches his legs.

Karen, age seventy-two, has been attending classes for ten years. After warming up with a cycle of Downward- and Upward-Facing Dog, she relaxes on the Backbender, a wooden support in the shape of a whale (see photo, page 7). Her fingers go all the way to the floor when she stretches her arms overhead.

Susan, age sixty-four, has just started kicking up into Handstands on her own. When she first came to yoga three years ago, she practiced Downward-Facing Dog with her hands on a chair, and she laughed when I told her that Handstands were within her reach. This morning she stretches briefly in Downward-Facing Dog Pose, and then kicks up lightly with the spunk and grace of a child.

Vivian, age sixty-seven, is sitting on the floor with her legs loosely crossed and is gently stretching her hips. She has practiced yoga for several years and has used it to cope with various health challenges, including cancer. At this time last year her head was bald from chemotherapy treatments, and her practice since has focused mainly on restorative poses to support her immune system and replenish her energy reserves.

Tom is hanging in the lower wall ropes in Downward-Facing Dog Pose. He is a runner, fifty-four years old, and says he doesn't really like yoga but his wife makes him come to class. He admits, however, with a sly smile, that he loves Hanging Dog Pose.

Students in my classes for older beginners generally range in age from forty-five up. Many arrive early so they can warm up with the wall ropes or relax with their legs up on the wall. A typical class will begin with a centering seated pose, such as

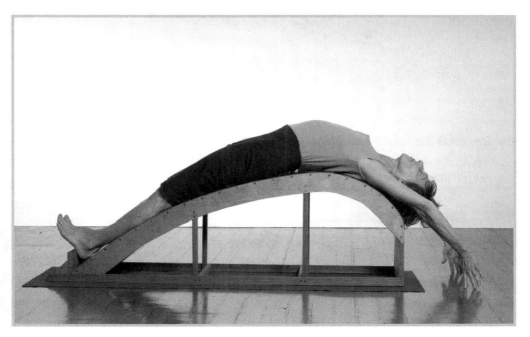

Lying on the Backbender opens the chest and increases blood flow to the heart.

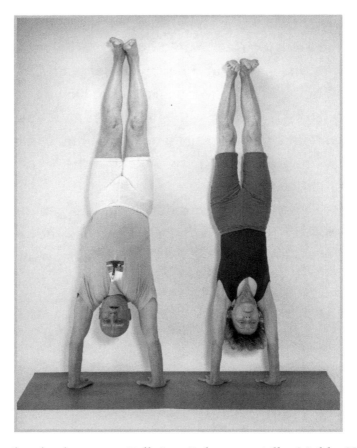

*Handstands, also known as Full Arm Balance or **Adho Mukha Vrkasana**, which means Downward-Facing Tree Pose in Sanskrit. Handstands are exhilarating and empowering.*

Bound-Angle Pose, or sitting with the legs crossed loosely, with the majority of the students sitting on two folded blankets or a bolster to help lengthen their spines and open their posture. Bent knee positions are generally followed by straight leg positions, such as sitting with the feet wide apart in Seated Wide-Angle Pose.

Almost every class includes Downward-Facing Dog Pose because it builds strength and flexibility in the upper body, stretches the legs, and has many of the benefits of inverted poses. Downward-Facing Dog Pose is followed by Upward-Facing Dog Pose. These two poses are often practiced with the hands on a chair seat, yoga blocks, or other support.

Standing poses are practiced with the support of props. Older beginners—especially if they have balance problems, arthritis, or osteoporosis—can practice standing poses with the back of the body near a wall, window sill, or other support, such as a yoga bar known as the *horse* or *trestle*, and with the bottom hand on a block, chair, or other support.

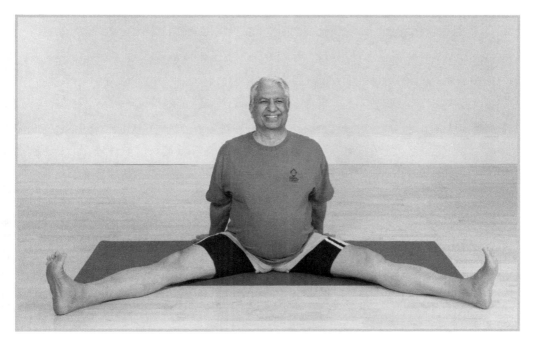

Seated Wide-Angle Pose, **Upavistha Konasana,** *helps you to enjoy sitting on the floor.*

New students also gain confidence by practicing with the back foot to the wall while holding onto a wall rope and a chair for extra support. Seated chair twists often follow standing poses.

The more experienced older students practice all the basic inverted poses, including Headstand and Shoulderstand, usually with the help of a wall or a chair. I expect my students who start in their fifties and sixties (and in some cases older) to gradually develop the strength to practice Right-Angle Handstand or Full Arm Balance at the wall.

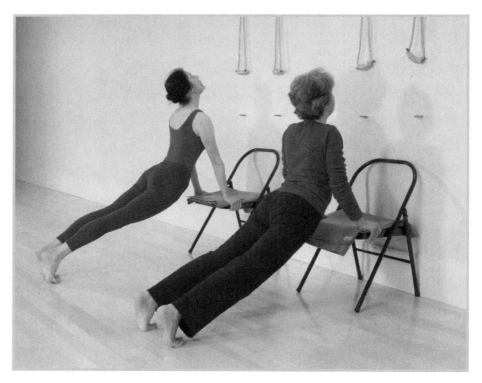

Upward-Facing Dog Pose, **Urdhva Mukha Svanasana,** *with the hands on a chair seat, helps to prepare the body for practicing the pose from the floor.*

A typical class also includes a variety of lying-down poses. These include Lying-Down Big-Toe Pose, and all the variations, with bolsters and other supports available to keep the back of the body level on the floor when students take their legs out to the side.

Classes end with deep relaxation in *Savasana*, the Corpse Pose. For older practitioners this pose has special meaning, as it helps them to face death and teaches the art of letting go (see Chapter 12, "The Last Asana").

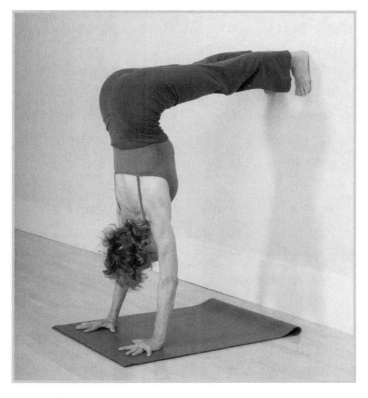

Right-Angle Handstand builds upper body strength. Notice how the head is below the level of the heart. My students of all ages enjoy practicing this energizing pose!

Yoga and the New Paradigm for Healthy Aging

Please forget about antiaging and avoid obsession with life extension. Instead, let's focus on preventing or minimizing the impact of age-related disease, on separating longevity and senescence, on learning how to live long and well, on how to age gracefully.

Andrew Weil, M.D., *Healthy Aging: A Lifelong Guide to Physical and Spiritual Well-Being*

Thanks to pioneers such as Dr. Andrew Weil, saying *healthy* and *aging* in the same breath is no longer considered a contradiction in terms. At the heart of healthy aging is the understanding that getting older is part of the nature of life, but we have many ways to help our minds and bodies to continue to function well. Dr. Weil highly recommends gentle, therapeutic forms of yoga for older people, and I was happy to see him balancing in Tree Pose on his website, www.healthyaging.com.

The old paradigm of the aging process has been one of ever-increasing stiffness, rigidity, and closing down, mentally and physically. Medical research on aging has clearly shown that without proper exercise, the body contracts and we lose height, strength, and flexibility. Our natural free range of motion becomes restricted, so daily activities become difficult and in some cases impossible.

Movement lubricates our muscles, ligaments, and joints. Stretching daily prevents stiffening, the first visible sign of premature aging. Yoga postures reverse the aging process by moving each joint in the body through its full range of motion—stretching, strengthening, and balancing each part.

Taking our joints through their full range of motion can help prevent degenerative arthritis or mitigate disability by massaging and lubricating cartilage and joints that normally aren't used. Joint cartilage is like a sponge; it receives fresh nutrients only when its fluid is squeezed out and a new supply can be soaked up. Without proper sustenance, neglected areas of cartilage can eventually wear out, exposing the underlying bone, like worn-out brake pads.

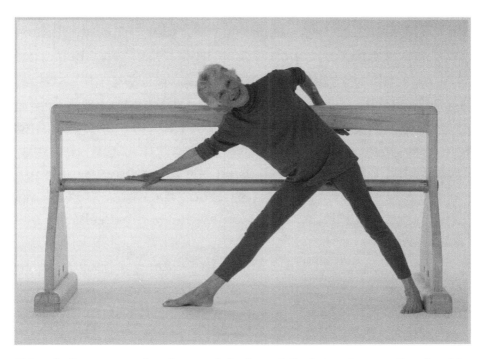

Triangle Pose, upper hand around the bar of the horse to open the shoulder joint.

Removing years of accumulated tightness and stiffness from your body feels like turning back the clock. Poses that initially seem impossible become possible as your whole body becomes more flexible. Most other forms of exercise contract muscles and tighten the body, which only adds to the stiffness that settles in with the passage of time. In our muscle-fitness–oriented culture, obsessed with outer appearance, we too often tighten the muscles to make the body look firmer. What is much more important, especially as we grow older, is opening and lengthening the body so that the aging process is tempered. In yoga, strength is balanced with youthful flexibility.

Yoga builds strength safely and incrementally. Strong, supple muscles help protect us as we grow older from conditions such as arthritis, osteoporosis, and back pain and help prevent falls. It's well documented that weight-bearing exercise strengthens bones and helps ward off osteoporosis. Many postures in yoga require that you lift your own weight. And some, such as Downward-Facing Dog Pose and Upward-Facing Dog Pose, help strengthen the arm bones, which are particularly vulnerable to osteoporotic fractures. This allows us to move more freely and to enjoy our bodies well into our later years.

While we cannot predict or control what happens to us in life, a yoga practice promotes inner strength and confidence in our ability to absorb inevitable stresses. A sense of inner well-being, not dependent on outside circumstances, promotes an attitude that helps us make better choices in all aspects of our lives.

*No other physical exercise can be
tailored to such widely-varied physical capabilities—
or limitations—of class attendees as does yoga.
It's non-threatening, has no side effects
and can be considered preventive care, and
in some cases, cure as well.*

Frank Iszak, founder, Silver Age Yoga

"You Are as Young as Your Spine Is Flexible"

The close relationship between yoga and aging begins with the spine. Yoga is unique in its capacity to prevent and even reverse the most conspicuous sign of aging—one that cannot be disguised or transformed cosmetically: the shortening and rounding of the spine.

Posture affects the health of every system of the body—not only the neuromuscular system (joints, bones and ligaments, muscles and tendons, and the nerves that move all of them) but also the endocrine system (pituitary, thyroid, adrenal and other glands) and the cardiovascular and respiratory systems. Lengthening the spine to create space between the vertebrae is vital to our health because nerves connected to the structures of the body, including the internal organs, branch out from the spinal cord between the vertebrae.

In adults, all nourishment to the spine comes from movement. Yoga nourishes the spinal disks: the shock absorbers between the vertebrae that can herniate and compress nerves. Without movement, the disks of the spine gradually shrink, which causes the body to lose height. Fluids are drawn into and flushed out of the disks by stretching, lengthening, and moving the spine in all directions: forward, backward, sideways, and twisting. If the disks are not nourished, they start to shrink and lose their elasticity, becoming more prone to the injury known as a "crush fracture."

In the modern world, people spend many hours each day engaged in work that tends to pull the upper body forward. A rounded back leads to a sunken chest, which causes shallow breathing and contributes to cardiovascular and other health problems. A rounded back, forward head and collapsed chest are so common that we almost consider them a normal part of growing older. Yoga counteracts and reverses all of this.

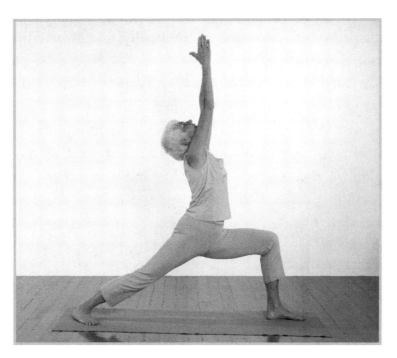

Warrior I, **Virabhadrasana I,** *strengthens and lengthens the spine.*

Maintaining the health and integrity of the spine is the central theme of yoga. Yoga develops spinal strength and agility, slowing and even reversing the common degenerative changes often found in people at midlife and older. In this book you will learn specific ways to protect your back from disk injuries and how to maintain the health of your spine for a lifetime.

Inverted Poses: Elixir of Life

Inverted poses are the heart of a yoga practice for people over fifty. They bring emotional balance and mental clarity, and—by improving the flow of blood to and from the heart—they refresh and rejuvenate the entire body.

Good circulation and good health are intimately connected. When the circulation of blood is restricted, the cells of our body do not get the oxygen and nutrients needed to function effectively. When our circulation is sluggish, our vital energy drops and our whole physical, emotional, and mental response to daily life tends to take a negative turn.

Yoga helps increase circulation, especially to our head, hands, and feet. Yoga also delivers more oxygen to our cells, which function better as a result. Twisting poses wring out venous blood from internal organs and allow fresh oxygenated blood to flow in once the twist is released. Inverted poses, such as Headstand, Handstand, and Shoulderstand, encourage venous blood from the legs and pelvis to flow back to the heart, where it can be pumped to the lungs to be freshly oxygenated.

Turning the body halfway or completely upside down increases the circulation to the upper body, including the brain. Blood circulates around the neck, chest, and head, helping the lungs, throat, and sinuses to become resistant to infection. The endocrine glands in the throat and head (thyroid and parathyroid glands) also benefit from improved circulation. Upside-down poses control the metabolism of the body and regulate blood pressure, glucose levels, and chemical balance.

The gravitational force of Earth is among the most powerful physical influences on the human body, and after the age of fifty it becomes increasingly important to reverse the downward pull of gravity on the body. In effect, inverted yoga positions

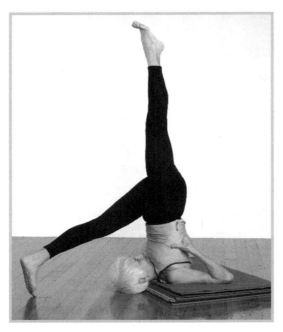

One-Legged Supported Shoulderstand, **Eka Pada Salamba Sarvangasana.**

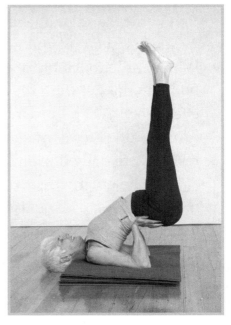

Shoulderstand variation, known as Inverted Lake Seal, **Viparita Karani Mudra.**

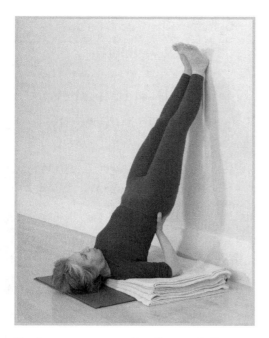 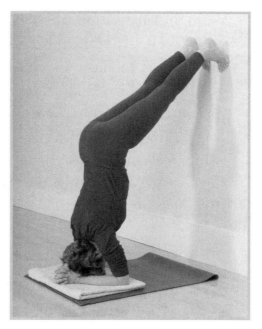

*Beginners can practice Supported
Shoulderstand and other inverted poses
with the help of a wall.*

Headstand at the wall.

turn gravity itself upside down and are thus among the best
means of slowing down and even reversing the aging process.

Due to cardiovascular problems related to aging, such as
arteriosclerosis (hardening of the arteries), blood flow to the
brain gradually decreases. Dr. Krishna Raman, in his writings
on yoga and the circulatory system, states that by the time a
person is age sixty-five, the blood flow to the brain may be
one-third of what it was at age twenty-five. The ravages of
senility are apparent in every nursing home in the country.
Western medicine accepts the fact that this is a degenerative
disease usually associated with inadequate circulation to the

brain, but it has found few ways of preventing or treating it. Yoga teaches that the most effective way of increasing blood to the brain is to allow gravity to do the work for you. Inverted positions, which bring the brain below the level of the heart, permit circulation to the upper body to increase without putting strain on the heart.

In addition to these benefits, yoga helps us on the path to healthy, graceful aging in other ways that are summarized in the following section.

Yoga is a gift for older people.
One who studies yoga in the later years
gains not only health and happiness, but also
freshness of mind since yoga gives one a bright outlook
on life. One can look forward to a more healthful
future rather than looking back into the past.
With yoga, a new life begins, even if started later.
Yoga is a rebirth which teaches one to face the rest of
one's life happily, peacefully and courageously.

Geeta S. Iyengar, *Yoga: A Gem for Women*

Gifts of Yoga for Graceful Aging

If you can breathe, you can do yoga. Yoga teaches us how to breathe deeply, without strain. The ability to positively affect your body's functioning through the way you breathe is recognized in many areas of modern medicine and daily life. The two top benefits of yoga breathing are its effectiveness in stress reduction and pain management. With few exceptions, yoga teaches us to breathe through our two nostrils, which is both calming and more efficient. When you breathe through your nose, the air is filtered (pollen and dirt are removed, which can help to protect against airborne diseases), and it is warmed and humidified (cold dry air is more likely to trigger an asthma attack in people who are sensitive).

Yoga reduces the need for prescription drugs. Studies of people with insomnia, asthma, high blood pressure, depression, heart conditions, Type II diabetes (formerly called *adult-onset diabetes*) and other diseases have shown that yoga helped them to reduce their dosage of medications and sometimes to taper off them entirely. Between ages fifty-five and sixty-five, individuals are typically given an average of eight different prescriptions during any given year. People older than seventy take an average of eight different medications daily. Older people have been known to take as many as thirty different medications during the last year of their lives. The U.S. Food and Drug Administration reports that the average older person takes two over-the-counter drugs daily in addition to prescription medications. Each year in the United States, medication problems are the cause of over 280,000 hospitalizations for people age sixty-five and older. Recent studies show a link between drug use and dizziness, loss of balance, falling, other accidents, Alzheimer's disease, and other dementia-related disorders.

Yoga can ease pain. According to several studies, breathing practices, yoga postures, relaxation techniques, and meditation reduced pain in people with arthritis, back pain, fibromyalgia, carpal tunnel syndrome, and other chronic conditions. Yoga helps break the vicious cycle of not moving due to chronic pain. When you relieve pain, your state of mind improves, you're more motivated to be active, and you reduce the need for pain or mood-altering medication.

Yoga reduces stress and boosts the immune system. Modern medicine points to stress as a major cause of disease. Normally, the adrenal glands secrete the stress hormone cortisol in response to an acute crisis, which temporarily boosts immune function. If your cortisol levels stay high even after the crisis has passed, this can compromise the immune system. Additionally, elevated levels of cortisol have been linked with depression, osteoporosis, high blood pressure, and insulin resistance.

Yoga helps calm your nervous system. Yoga encourages you to relax, slow down your breathing, and focus on the present moment. This contributes to what Dr. Herbert Benson calls the *relaxation response*—lower breathing and heart rates, decreased blood pressure, and increased blood flow to the intestines and reproductive organs.

Yoga helps to release chronic tension. Gripping the steering wheel in traffic jams, tensing your neck and shoulders while on the computer, chronic anxiety over unpaid bills, and unresolved relationship issues can lead to a vicious cycle of chronic tension that further increases stress and darkens our mood. Yoga helps to break this cycle.

Yoga results in fewer stress-related health problems. Ulcers, irritable bowel syndrome, constipation—all can be exacerbated by stress. Yogis through the ages have observed that inverted and twisting poses are especially beneficial in getting waste to move through the system. When we practice yoga, we become more aware of where we hold chronic, habitual tension and how to let go and release it. We cannot control what happens in life—but we can choose, to a far greater extent than we realize, how we respond.

Yoga is good for your heart. Studies have found that yoga practice lowers the resting heart rate, increases endurance, and can improve your maximum uptake of oxygen during exercise—all reflections of improved aerobic conditioning.

Yoga helps balance your blood pressure. Two studies of people with hypertension compared the effects of *Savasana* (Corpse Pose) to lying passively on a couch. After three months, *Savasana* was associated with a drop of twenty-six points in systolic blood pressure (the top number) and a drop of fifteen points in diastolic blood pressure (the bottom number). In addition, the higher the initial blood pressure, the bigger the drop.

Yoga helps balance blood sugar. Yoga lowers blood sugar. It also lowers low-density lipoprotein (LDL, also known as "bad" cholesterol) and boosts high-density lipoprotein (HDL, or "good" cholesterol) in the blood. In people with diabetes, yoga has been found to lower blood sugar in several ways: by lowering cortisol and adrenaline levels, by encouraging weight loss, and by improving sensitivity to the effects of insulin. Get your blood-sugar levels down, and you decrease your risk of diabetic complications such as heart attack, kidney failure, and blindness.

Yoga sharpens your mind. An integral part of yoga is learning how to be in the present. Studies have found that regular yoga practice improves coordination, reaction time, memory, and even IQ scores.

Yoga improves your balance. Practicing yoga regularly increases proprioception (the ability to feel what your body is doing and where it is in space) and improves balance. For those of us who are older, this translates into more independence and delayed admission to an assisted living home—or possibly never entering one at all. Balance poses such as Tree Pose and other standing poses can make us feel more steady on our feet.

Yoga promotes deeper, more restful sleep. Studies suggest that another by-product of a regular yoga practice is better sleep, which means feeling less tired, less stressed, more clear-headed, and less likely to have accidents. An estimated two-thirds of Americans have a sleep-related problem. One study found that building up a sleep deficit adversely affects carbohydrate metabolism and the functioning of the endocrine glands, such as the thyroid. The effects are similar to those seen in normal aging, which means that sleep debt may increase the severity of age-related chronic disorders.

Yoga lifts your spirits. Studies find that a consistent yoga practice reduced depression and led to a significant increase in serotonin levels and a decrease in the levels of cortisol and monoamine oxidase (an enzyme that breaks down neurotransmitters). At the University of Wisconsin, Richard Davidson, Ph.D., found that the left prefrontal cortex showed heightened activity in people who meditate, a finding that has been correlated with greater levels of happiness and better immune function.

It is well established that many older people suffer from depression. In a series of studies, Dr. David Shapiro, a physician at the UCLA Department of Psychiatry, has examined the link between physical movements, posture, and emotion. Dr. Shapiro, who is a practitioner of Iyengar yoga, estimates that as many as 1 million Americans begin yoga as a means to alleviate depression. He hypothesized that stretching and pressure at reflex points on the skin affects functions of the organs and glands and that specific postures may have an effect on emotional release. In "Mood Changes Associated with Iyengar Yoga Practices," one of his studies, he compared classes that emphasized either forward bends, standing poses, or backbends and found a reduction in negative moods for all three types of classes and a significant increase in positive emotions for classes that focused mainly on backbends.

As yoga becomes more prevalent as a complementary therapy that appears to achieve positive results, studies such as those cited in this chapter and throughout this book will be increasing. The International Association of Yoga Therapists (IAYT), listed in Appendix C, has compiled an extensive bibliography of research and resources on yoga and seniors by doctors, yoga teachers, gerontologists, and other health professionals. This bibliography, as well as a broad spectrum of other information on yoga and healthy aging, is available on the IAYT website, www.iayt.org.

BETTY EILER

After Seventy, Include Yoga in Your Lifestyle!

A Day in the Yoga Life of Betty Eiler

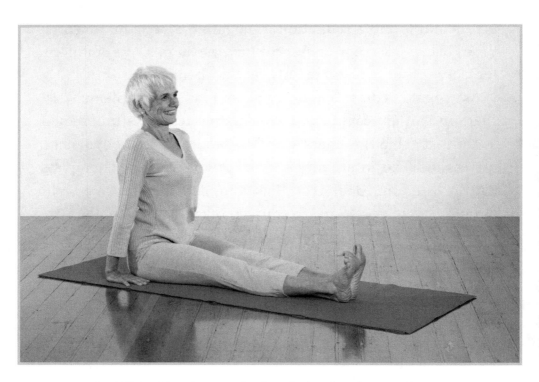

*Staff Pose, **Dandasana**, the foundation for the seated pose.*

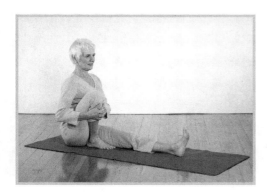

Preparation, one knee bent.

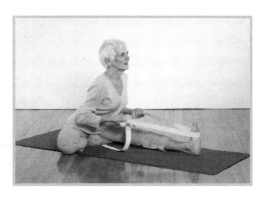

Head to Knee Pose, **Janusirsasana,** *with strap.*

Head to Knee Pose, a restful variation with the head supported.

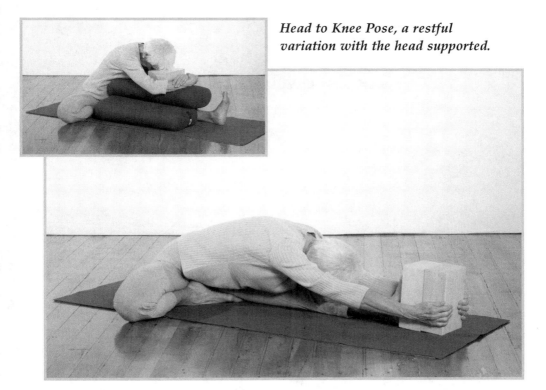

Head to Knee Pose, hands extending past the feet, holding blocks. This asana tones the liver and the spleen, and thereby aids digestion. It also tones and activates the kidneys.

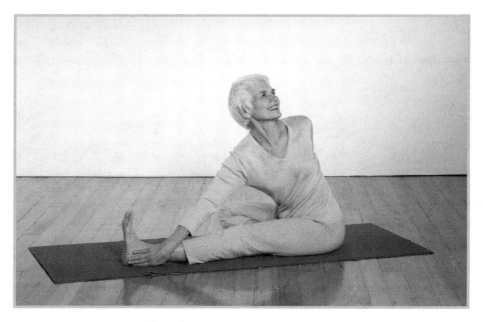

Head to the Knee Pose, twist variation.

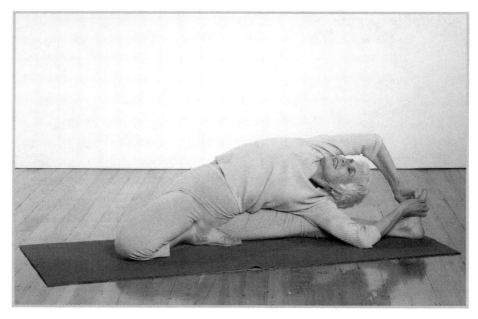

Revolved Head to Knee Pose, **Parivritta Janusirsasana,** *a joyous, heart-opening pose.*

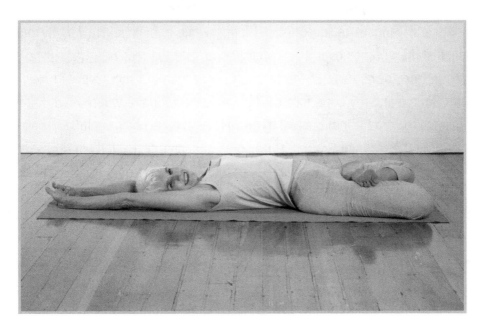

Lying-Down Lotus Pose, **Supta Padmasana.**

*B*etty Eiler was born on November 22, 1934. She and Barbara
Wiechmann (whose story follows) met in 1987 at the Ramamani
Memorial Institute in India when they traveled to India to study with
B. K. S. Iyengar and Geeta Iyengar.

Betty and Barbara are both longtime students of Ramanand Patel. Betty
currently divides her time between Mexico and California. She has played
many roles in life, but she says her favorite role is that of mother of four
children.

Betty believes that yoga cannot protect us from the trials and tribula-
tions of life, but our practice can help us cope with whatever challenges
life brings us. To illustrate this point she told me the following story:

My son (Rogge) received a head injury while in college. He was in four rehabilitation homes over a two-year period, and the recovery was a whole new journey of its own. Living through it with him put me deeper in touch with Source and my core beliefs. There was even a point where I felt that if I needed to care for him the rest of my life, I would still be grateful. That was a profound awakening for me. Gifts come in such unexpected packages!

Now that I'm in my seventies, my practice is less structured than it was previously. My hours of waking and sleeping vary, as do my eating habits. I eat small meals according to the requests of my body. My interests, personal goals, family, and consciousness guide my life flow, and yoga has inherently become part of that flow. My yoga varies as each day, each week, and each month vary.

Some days, I feel the need for a deep, long, vigorous practice centered around standing poses, inversions, a few backbends, and then *Savasana*. Other days, after playing tennis, I prefer to do more sitting poses with leg stretches, hip openers, a few twists, and forward bends.

Then again, there are times when I have a full day of other activities and I do yoga postures around what I am doing, so there is no particular period of practice. This kind of practice could be compared to eating several small meals a day depending on what the body wants.

At age seventy-one I am growing wrinkles, feeling more sensitive, and experiencing the weathering of time. I feel very healthy. I attribute my good health to yoga, *Ayurveda*, and nutritional supplements. I am deeply grateful for the wisdom of the great teachers who brought us natural healing, for the wisdom of modern-day scientific research on nutrition, and especially for the knowledge of the ancient science of yoga.

BARBARA WIECHMANN
How I Discovered Yoga in the Haight-Ashbury

A Day in the Yoga Life of Barbara Wiechmann

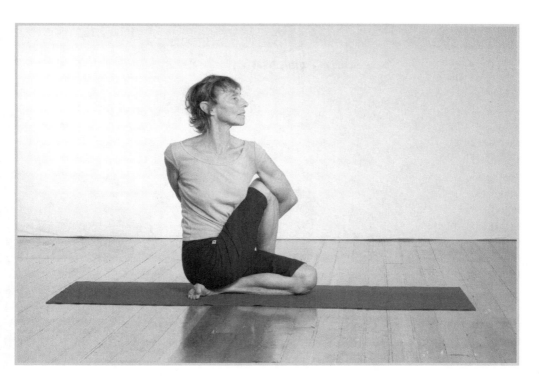

Seated Twist, **Marichyasana IV.**
Spinal twists massage and tone your abdominal organs.

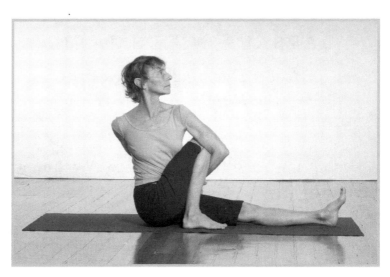

Seated Twist, **Marichyasana III.**

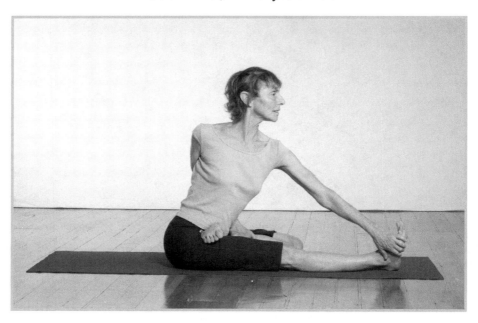

Half-Bound Lotus Forward Bend Pose, **Ardha Baddha Padma Paschimottanasana.**
Seated poses elongate the spine and alleviate stiffness in the ankles, knees, hips and groins, giving the body the strength and flexibility it needs to sit quietly in meditation.

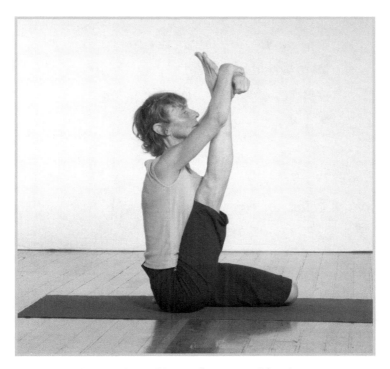

Heron Pose, **Krounchasana,** *side view.*

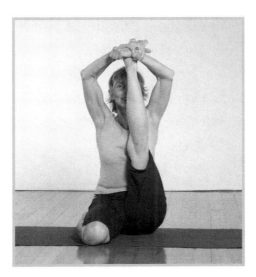

Heron Pose, **Krounchasana,** *front view.*

*Doing yoga over the
last three decades has been like living
in an eternally blooming flower.*

Barbara Wiechmann

*B*arbara Wiechmann enjoys practicing with her longtime friend
Betty Eiler.

We both love yoga so much, it brought us together and made sisters out
of us. Our lives often take us in different directions, but when we get together
there is an instant closeness as if no time or miles have ever separated us.

*Barbara is the proud mother of three sons and grandmother of three
girls. Her favorite pastimes include hanging out with her children and
grandchildren, walking, reading, listening to music, and dancing the
Argentine tango. About yoga, she says this:*

It's an ongoing miracle in my life—a gift that I am incredibly grateful to
have been given and even more delighted to be able to share.

*Barbara's emphasis when teaching is on helping students feel the
joyful, liberating aspect of yoga in the belief that this liberation frees
the student to find and express his or her true nature and potential.*

*Here, in her own words, is the story of how Barbara first discovered
yoga.*

This is the story of how yoga found me! I had moved into a flat in the Haight-Ashbury (San Francisco) with a friend of mine. When we moved in, there was a picture of a yogi in *Simhasana* (Lion Pose) on the wall of the bathroom. We thought it was very amusing and left the picture up. One afternoon, a few weeks later, the doorbell rang. I opened the door, and there on the doorstep was a very handsome man with long, flowing hair. He was bare chested and wore loose-fitting white cotton pants. His feet were also bare. He carried a skateboard.

I frowned, being rather suspicious of this strange, half-naked man on my doorstep. He explained that he had been skateboarding down my street when he fell off his skateboard and stubbed his toe.

"May I please use your bathroom to wash my foot?" he asked. How could I say no? Once in my bathroom he saw the picture of *Simhasana* on the wall and said, "Oh, you do yoga!" I replied that actually I didn't but had long wanted to learn. (It was very hard to find yoga teachers in those days.) Then, as in a fairy tale, he said, "I am a yoga teacher. I teach at Shire School (one of the first alternative schools in San Francisco). I would be happy to give you a free yoga lesson."

Well, I took him up on it and loved the first class. His first name was Eric (I am not sure if I ever learned his last name). Once a week for a year he came to our flat and gave my roommate and me a private lesson. He charged us only a dollar each per class! After about a year, he left for Switzerland. I never saw him again! Eric, wherever you are, THANK YOU!!!

CHAPTER 2

Yoga and Yoga Props:
Lifelines for the Later Years

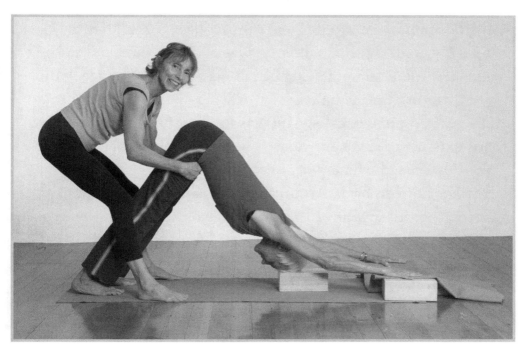

Downward-Facing Dog Pose, **Adho Mukha Svanasana,** *with the hands and forehead supported by yoga blocks. Practicing with a partner helps you learn to stretch your hips back and elongate your spine.*

*The use of props is the single distinct
advantage that the system of Iyengar Yoga offers.
It has provided a very effective way to practice every pose
without strain or error, and has thus carved for
itself a special niche in the field of the
medical applications of yoga.*

Krishna Raman, M.D., *A Matter of Health*

At the age of eighty-seven, Iyengar joked that he invented props when he was a young man so that he could still practice yoga in his old age. I still recall the words of my first yoga teacher, nearing sixty, telling me that she started yoga because she was looking for "exercise without exhaustion." When we are young, the physical energy of youth seems inexhaustible. Even if we wear ourselves out, we quickly bounce back. Around midlife, sometimes sooner, we become more aware of the depletion of our natural energy reserves. Our bodies begin to show signs of wear and tear. While the natural aging process cannot be halted, yoga offers a way to slow it down, conserve health, and rebuild our precious energy reserves.

Yoga is the art and science of spiritual, mental, and physical transformation. It is a classical Indian discipline that is as relevant in the twenty-first century as it was when it was developed thousands of years ago. Yoga is a nonviolent way of life that encourages each individual to feel whole and to realize his or her inner potential.

The word *yoga* comes from a Sanskrit root that means *yoke, join, unite,* or *make whole*. This ancient discipline cultivates the union between individual and universal consciousness.

The exact origins of yoga are uncertain, but its practices and principles predate written history. In the Indus Valley (now Pakistan), archaeologists have uncovered 5,000-year-old carvings of adepts in yoga positions. The science of yoga was originally passed down orally from teacher to student and was codified in written form about 2,000 years ago. The *Yoga Sutras*, by Patanjali, form the foundation upon which the structure of yoga has been built.

Yoga is not a religion, but its teachings have been influenced by various religions, traditions, and sacred scriptures. Ancient texts present holistic views that encompass the physical, mental, and spiritual dimensions of the practitioner. Over the ages, different forms of yoga have emerged to blend with particular philosophical and religious beliefs practiced by the people of those times and places. Today, millions of people worldwide practice many diversified yoga styles that stem from a common ancient source.

Yoga Asanas: Practical Tools for Life

A yoga pose is known by the Sanskrit term *asana*. The terms, *pose, asana,* and *posture* are used interchangeably in this book. *Asana* is the positioning of the body in various standing, lying-down, upside-down, or seated postures. Asanas are one of yoga's most significant and practical tools for integrating all aspects of a human being—body, mind, and spirit.

The word *healing* comes from the root "to make whole." Among the many health benefits that set yoga apart from other forms of physical exercise is the effect that yoga postures and breathing practices have on the vitality of our organs and glands. This book describes the effect that asanas have on all the systems of the body. Yoga's inverted poses are particularly important in the later years as they have a powerful effect on the neuroendocrine system by allowing fresh, oxygenated blood to flow to the glands in the head and neck.

According to Iyengar, "In each asana, different organs are placed in different anatomical positions, and are squeezed and spread, dampened and dried, heated and cooled. The organs are supplied with fresh blood and are gently massaged, relaxed, and toned into a state of optimum health." (See *Yoga: The Path to Holistic Health* in Appendix D).

Iyengar Yoga and Yoga Props

B. K. S. Iyengar is widely credited with the development of practicing yoga with the help of props. Although the use of props was known earlier in crude form, Iyengar evolved both their use and the sequences of asanas commonly practiced today. He categorized groups of poses according to anatomical structure, physiological functioning and psychological effect.

Iyengar's early writings describe how he began experimenting with ordinary, everyday objects such as walls, chairs, stools, blocks, bolsters, blankets, and belts to help his students move deeper into postures. By providing more height, weight, and support, he discovered that props helped students of all ages and all levels understand and retain key movements and subtle adjustments of the body. These discoveries inspired him to experiment further and to create props adjusted to suit individual needs.

Today the therapeutic use of props for special populations is one of the most distinguishing features of Iyengar yoga and one that many other schools (styles) of yoga are integrating into their curriculum. Iyengar's innovations in the understanding, practice, and teachings of yoga are described in great detail in his books and videos. *Yoga: The Path to Holistic Health* illustrates the use of sequences of poses supported with props to treat or prevent over eighty ailments. Iyengar demystified what had previously been a somewhat secret, exclusive, and inaccessible art. He made yoga immensely practical and accessible to ordinary men and women, including those who begin in the later years.

What Are Props and Why Do We Use Them?

In the world of yoga, a prop is any object that provides height, weight, or support and helps you stretch, strengthen, balance, relax, or improve your body alignment. Props are used both for therapeutic purposes, as previously mentioned, and to teach specific actions such as "lifting the kneecaps," "elongating the spine," "opening the chest," and others, which you will hear repeated over and over again in yoga classes.

Props also help you stay in poses for a longer time and conserve your energy, allowing the nervous system to relax. They can be used to make postures more challenging; to safely stretch farther; to work in a deeper, stronger way; and to expand, open, and blossom in a pose. In yoga we are asking the body to "work against the grain." We are asking the body to let go of the death grip that habit and conditioning have on us. Props help us to accept this revolutionary (and evolutionary) process.

Props include sticky mats (also referred to as "yoga mats"), blankets, belts, blocks, benches, wall ropes, sandbags, chairs, and other objects that help students experience the various yoga poses more profoundly. The ancient yogis used wood logs, stones, and ropes to help their practice. Many common features of our homes can also serve as props: floors, walls, corners, doors, doorways, hallways, stairs, ledges, windowsills, kitchen counters, even the kitchen sink!

Using yoga props makes postures safer and more accessible. Most older people are quite stiff by the time they start yoga, and props allow them to practice poses they would not ordinarily be able to do. Older students also frequently come to yoga with problems, ranging from back and neck pain to knee problems to old injuries. The more problems a student has, the more useful yoga props are.

Props allow you to hold poses longer, so you can experience their healing effects. By supporting the body in the yoga posture, muscles can lengthen in a passive, nonstrenuous way. By opening the body, the use of props also helps to improve blood circulation and breathing capacity.

For example, if you are unable to bend forward and bring your hands to the floor without straining, you can place your hands on a chair or wall. As the backs of your legs become more flexible, you will find that you can put your hands on a lower prop, such as a bench or a block. Props can still be used when the student wants to practice the pose in a more restorative way, even though he or she is capable of practicing the pose independently.

Supporting the body with props opens the door to *restorative yoga*, which not only allows you to exercise without exerting any effort but simultaneously relaxes and reenergizes you. This is critical during times when we find ourselves feeling too tired to exercise and then feeling even more tired because we are *not* exercising.

The creative use of props expands the help a teacher can give, especially when teaching a class with students of various levels of ability. For example, students who are not strong enough to practice inversions on their own can safely do so supported by ropes suspended from the wall or ceiling. In this way inversions can be performed without strain, and the student can receive the benefits of the pose.

Props are also used to teach students how a pose done correctly should feel. A rope hanging from a wall hook or doorknob and placed at the top of the legs in Downward-Facing Dog Pose, *Adho Mukha Svanasana*, allows the student to stretch the torso and arms as far forward as possible. Because the rope pulls the student's weight back into the legs, it helps the student experience the elongation of the abdomen and the deep muscles of the torso in the pose. The head can rest on a

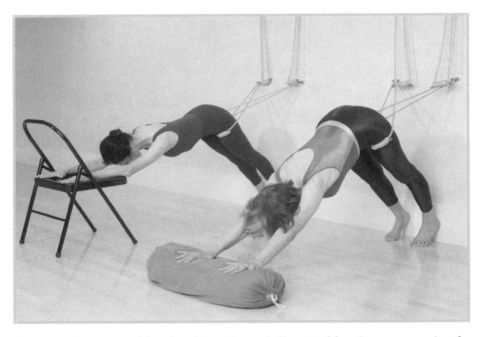

Hanging Downward-Facing Dog Pose, **Adho Mukha Svanasana,** *in the ropes. Props bring the weight of the pose into your hips and legs and remove pressure on your arms and shoulders.*

bolster or pillow. In this way, a wonderful, passive stretch is experienced. The student gets a taste of what it feels like to let go in a pose, to relax, and enjoy it. The use of props facilitates imprinting of the correct action in the pose so that the student understands it when the prop has been removed.

By using props, students who need to conserve their energy can practice more strenuous poses without overexerting themselves. People with chronic illness can use props to practice without undue strain and fatigue.

Props are adapted to each student's body type and flexibility. They are especially helpful to anyone who may avoid certain poses because of fear, problems with balance due to loss of hearing and eyesight, pain, or other limitations. In therapeutic situations, props are invaluable. People who have scoliosis (curvature of the spine), rounded back, or other chronic postural problems can significantly improve their posture by stretching with the help of a prop.

Iyengar introduced props into the modern practice of yoga to allow all practitioners access to the benefits of the postures regardless of physical condition, age, or length of study. He also explored in depth how these modified poses could help people recover from illness or injury or psychological trauma. Iyengar and his teachers have worked with Western doctors with great success in the fields of heart and immune disease and spinal and orthopedic problems. *Props help all practitioners—including both the most advanced students and those of advanced years—to receive the deep benefits of postures held for sustained periods of time.*

Eight Reasons Why Props Are Beneficial for Older Practitioners

1. Props help us conserve and replenish energy, which becomes increasingly important as we grow older and also during times of illness.

2. Props make difficult poses more accessible and safe. They allow even those who start late in life to hold poses for a long time, without strain.

3. Props help prevent injuries and help old injuries to heal.

B. K. S. Iyengar on Using Props

B. K. S. Iyengar asserts that very few people make use of the last phase of life in a fruitful, useful way.

It is an art to check the aging process. To stop its ascendance, one should learn to make old age a useful weapon. In this stage of life, one becomes negative. Courage starts declining and intelligence becomes dull. Anxiety encircles the older person. Laziness becomes a part of old age.

Some in old age realize the importance of yoga and come for help. They have not done any yogic practice before and want to learn and do something; yet they are unable to do the yoga postures. At that state, the profound utility of props and their values are realized. Even incapable persons will find hope of doing something that keeps life flowing with joy.

Iyengar believes that students who come to yoga late in life have the advantage of keeping themselves fit, physically and mentally, using props. His experience has been that bolsters, chairs, backbending and other benches, wall ropes, and other props are useful in old age, when people may not be able to do the posture independently. He believes that props free the older student from anxiety:

Practice on props leads one toward non-attachment of the body. The brain calms down and sound sleep, a dream for many old people, comes naturally through the use of props.

4. People tend to stretch from their more flexible areas and rely on their better-developed muscles for strength. Props encourage weak parts to strengthen and stiff areas to stretch, thus balancing and realigning the whole body.

5. Props allow us to stay in poses long enough to release tension and experience deeper levels of relaxation.

6. Props help create space in the spine and in the joints, ever more important as we grow older and cope with issues such as osteoporosis, arthritis, and joint replacements.

7. Props allow older practitioners with balance problems to practice the weight-bearing standing poses, helping them to remain independent and out of wheelchairs.

8. Props allow us to practice inverted poses safely and to reverse the downward pull of gravity, slowing down the aging process.

Yoga Props: An Investment in Your Health

Sometimes when I teach in a private home, I'm dismayed to discover the student has buried her bolster or blankets in the closet where they are hard to reach. Do not hide your props out of sight! Props serve as reminders to practice. When I walk in the door and see my bolster waiting, already set up by the wall, I am much more apt to practice Supported Legs Up the Wall Pose, *Viparita Karani*, followed naturally by a series of refreshing end-of-the-day poses. When you are tired, get in the habit of lying on your bolster and relaxing deeply, instead of habitually flopping on the couch, eating, and watching TV.

Make it a priority to have some bare wall space so that you do not have to move furniture or take down paintings to practice inverted or standing poses at the wall. As long as there is space for a mat, you can do a well-rounded sequence of poses, even in limited space.

The following sections contain descriptions of the most frequently utilized props.

Yoga Mats. A sticky, nonskid yoga mat is essential for creating stability and preventing your hands and feet from slipping. The beauty of a mat is twofold: It provides a nonslippery surface, and it clears a space, both physically and psychologically, in which you can do your practice. I recommend that you make a space in your home to do yoga, or even dedicate an entire room. To my way of thinking, a dedicated yoga room is more important than a TV room or a guest room!

If you don't already have one, invest in one or two good-quality nonskid yoga mats. A standard mat is twenty-four inches wide, sixty-eight inches long, and approximately one-eighth of an inch thick. Longer mats are available for tall people. I find that many of my older students appreciate the extra padding of a thicker mat or two standard mats placed one on top of the other. Please note that a soft, mushy mat does not work. It is essential that the mat provide a firm, level surface.

A yoga mat is not just for standing on or to keep your hands from slipping. A mat can be rolled and placed behind the knees to open the joint. It can be folded and placed underneath the heel of the back foot to help create stability in standing poses. It can be used as extra padding under the heels of the hands to ease stiff, painful wrists.

I highly recommend having one good-quality, thicker nonskid mat and an extra lighter mat that is easy to fold for extra support in various postures and for traveling or practicing away from home.

Wool or Cotton Blankets. Blankets are mainly used to provide padding, lift, and support. As you will learn in the chapters on arthritis, osteoporosis, and hip problems, folded blankets are invaluable for maintaining the alignment of the pelvis and spine in seated poses. They are also used to create a stable platform to protect the neck from injury when practicing Shoulderstand and Plow Pose. In addition, if you have four to eight blankets and are adept at folding them, they can substitute for bolsters in supported backbends, inversions such as *Viparita Karani,* and other restorative poses.

Yoga Bolsters. Yoga bolsters are firm cushions that come in various shapes and sizes. They are used mainly to lift and support the body to promote deep, effortless relaxation in passive, restorative postures.

For the restorative poses shown in this book, I recommend a firm, round bolster stuffed with dense cotton so that you feel no sinking sensation when you lie on it. I want to emphasize that soft cushions or other material that the body sinks into do not have the desired effect. The best alternative is two or more blankets folded in the shape of a bolster. In some poses, blocks or a combination of blocks and blankets, or a rolled up yoga mat, can substitute.

While the width and height of the yoga bolster may vary, what makes it effective is the firm support it provides for the entire length of your spinal column. The muscles of your abdomen, chest, and back release their tension, lengthen, and relax deeply.

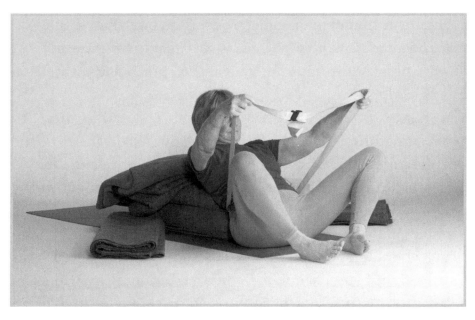

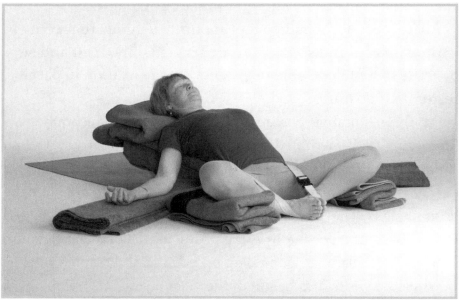

A bolster, folded blankets, and a strap help make the Supported Lying-Down Bound-Angle Pose, **Supta Baddha Konasana,** *sublimely comfortable and relaxing.*

Yoga bolsters are specifically designed so that the sides of your rib cage open and expand over the bolster and move downward toward the floor. When your rib cage expands laterally in this manner, your breathing capacity deepens naturally. The bolster leaves a vital, lasting impression on the body of what it feels like to have the chest open and free. Using the bolster enhances your awareness of your breath, as well as your ability to regulate and deepen your inhalations and exhalations.

I highly recommend obtaining one or two large, firm bolsters from a yoga prop company or yoga center.

Yoga Blocks. Blocks are useful for a wide variety of poses, especially for standing poses, where they support your hand and help keep the legs and spine in alignment. Two blocks under the hands are useful for practicing Downward- and Upward-Facing Dog and other poses. A single block has three alternate heights and shapes and can be used alone, stacked, or in a variety of different arrangements.

Yoga blocks are made from a variety of materials, including lightweight foam. Purchase blocks in sets so that they are identical in size and shape for poses that require a pair of blocks. You can get along nicely with one set of heavier, firmer, more stable wooden blocks, but as you practice you will discover poses where it is easier to work with a softer, slightly yielding surface and a lighter-weight block.

Gripitz: A Unique Set of Yoga Blocks. Gripitz are a pair of lightweight ergonomic blocks designed to be grasped by their handles. They help to relieve wrist strain in poses that require weight bearing on the hands, wrists, and arms, such as Downward-Facing Dog Pose and Upward-Facing Dog Pose.

Poses that require upper-body weight bearing are often painful for people with wrist problems. Blocks, wedges (see Wedges), and folded yoga mats are also helpful in relieving wrist strain.

Gripitz provide many of the benefits of a conventional block with some added features. The comfortable handles can be gripped, keeping the wrists straight rather than flexed. Practicing with them removes strain in the wrists while still allowing the bones and muscles of the arms to become stronger. One of my seventy-four-year-old students got such great results that she gave sets of them as gifts to others with wrist problems.

Gripitz handles also keep the hands from sliding, as can happen when using ordinary blocks. The handles are padded

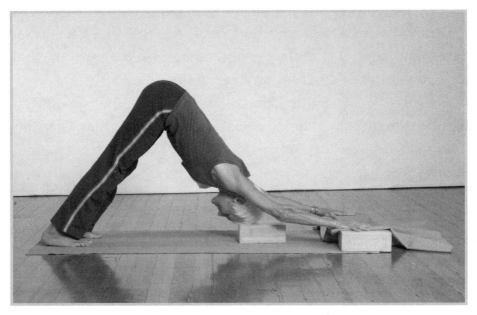

Downward-Facing Dog Pose, **Adho Mukha Svanasana.** *Placing your hands on blocks takes strain off the wrists and shoulder joints. Resting your forehead on a block or bolster is calming to the mind.*

with thin foam, making them comfortable to grip. The props are multipurpose and can also be used under the legs in restorative poses.

Wedges. A wedge or slant board made out of foam or wood can also be placed under the hands to reduce pressure on wrists. A folded yoga mat can serve a similar purpose. Wedges are also used to help anchor the heels.

Yoga Straps and Belts. A yoga strap is six- to ten-feet long and is used in dozens of innovative ways in seated, lying-down, inverted, standing, and backbending poses. Yoga straps, or belts, help prevent muscle and joint strain; keep

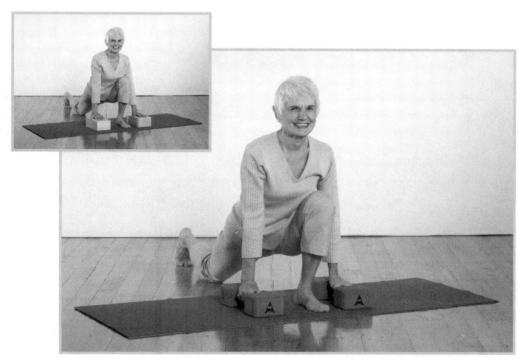

Lunge Pose. Blocks and Gripitz help remove wrist strain in a wide range of poses.

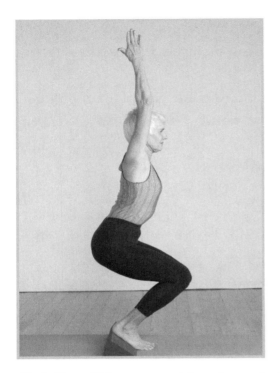

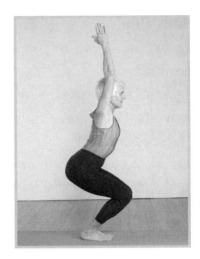

Chair Pose, **Utkatasana.**

Chair Pose, **Utkatasana,** *with wedge under heels,*
for those who cannot get their heels to the floor.

elbows, knees, and other body parts from splaying out; and enhance our overall ability to stretch without sacrificing good alignment. Straps make seemingly impossible stretching movements safe and possible, especially for older practitioners. For some poses, like lying-down leg stretches, you can substitute any soft belt or strap, but for most poses a real yoga strap with a buckle is much more convenient. The six-foot length is adequate for most basic positions, but if you are taller or larger you may need a longer strap. The longer straps are more versatile, and I recommend them highly. Examples of how to use straps are shown throughout the book.

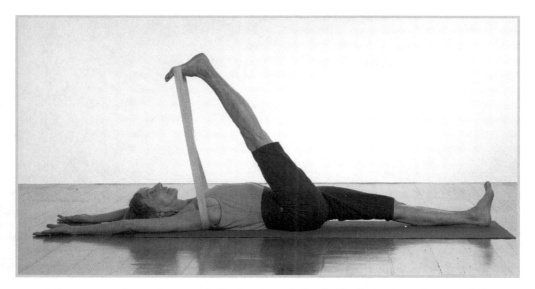

A long strap looped around the back and the ball of the foot is one of the most relaxing ways to stretch your hamstrings.

Sandbags and Other Weights. A yoga sandbag weighs ten pounds and is used to apply pressure to various areas of the body. One or more properly placed sandbags promote a deep sense of physical and psychological release. For example, a sandbag across the lower abdomen in Deep Relaxation Pose, or balanced on the soles of the feet in Supported Legs Up the Wall Pose, adds immensely to the depth of relaxation. When you first place the sandbag on your body you may be aware of the weight, but after a few breaths your body surrenders and it seems to disappear. Sandbags, as well as other properly placed weights, can also be used to promote circulation to specific areas and to increase the stretch in many poses. Sandbags and other weights are especially therapeutic during times of great stress when someone may have exceptional difficulty relaxing on their own.

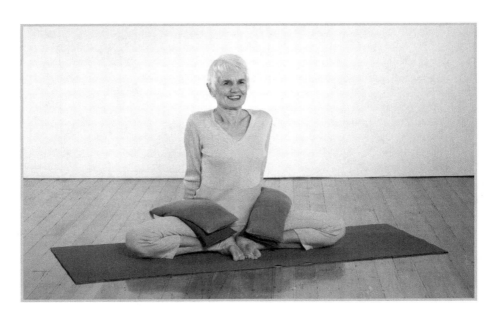

Bound-Angle Pose, **Baddha Konasana,** *practiced with sandbags, increases flexibility in the legs, hips, and lower back. Sandbags weigh ten pounds each. If you are new to yoga, start with one sandbag on each thigh.*

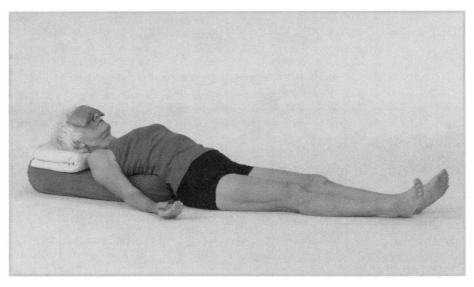

Supported Deep Relaxation Pose, Corpse Pose, **Savasana,** *practiced with a bolster and an eye bag.*

Eye Bags. Placing an eye bag (or eye pillow) over your eyes will help you relax more deeply. The gentle pressure helps quiet the mind by relaxing the muscles around your eyes, calming the involuntary movements of your eyes, creating darkness and removing visual stimuli. When selecting an eye bag, check that it is filled with flax seeds or other material that provides weight. Some people enjoy lightly scented eye bags, but it is the weight, not just the scent, that helps the eyes and brain to relax.

Suza's Secret Relaxation Tip

Store your eye bag in a clear freezer bag in the freezer. The coolness of the cold eye bag is extra relaxing. I have an eye bag filled with flax seed that is almost the size of a sandbag. It wraps around my head and covers my forehead and eyes. If I ever feel a headache coming on I practice Viparita Karani *for half an hour or longer with the ice-cold eye bag wrapped around my forehead and temples. You can also place two or three standard-size eye bags across your eyes and forehead.*

Chapters 4 and 5 and photographs throughout this book describe other props that are especially useful for older practitioners: walls, chairs, ropes, Backbenders (including the backbending bench), and the largest of the yoga props: a sturdy wooden yoga bar known as the horse, pony, trestle or tressler.

BERNARD SPIRA

Yoga at 94

*Every day you must walk that fine line
between courage and caution.*

B. K. S. Iyengar

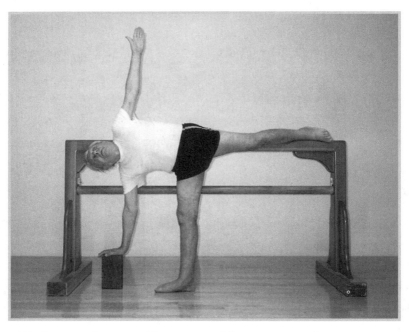

*Bernard Spira practices standing poses with a yoga prop known as
the* **horse, pony, tressler, or trestle.** *Similar to a thick, sturdier version of a
ballet bar, this large wooden prop allows standing poses to be practiced in a
way that creates precise alignment, stability, and balance. The horse conserves precious energy reserves, which becomes increasingly important as
we grow older.*

*The best thing I can do for myself is
hang upside down for five minutes.
I hang as long as I can so the
blood can go to my head.*

Bernard Spira

*W*hile reading the "Event Book" about B. K. S. Iyengar's **Light on Life** *book tour in southern California, I spotted an announcement that proclaimed, "Yoga at 92: The Bernard Spira Story." Underneath this headline was a photo of a nice-looking white-haired gentleman in a T-shirt and shorts practicing Warrior II (Virabhadrasana II). His arms and back were supported by a yoga horse. The photo caption read, "To Guruji B. K. S. Iyengar who has made all this possible. Thank you." Below the photo appeared Bernard's birth date, October 12, 1911, as well as a website: www.senioryogis.org.*

"Wow!" I said to myself. "This guy is serious!" I realized that here was a senior yogi whose experience deserved a wider audience. When I looked at www.senioryogis.com, one of the first images I saw was a photo of Bernard hanging upside down from a pelvic sling.

My curiosity was definitely piqued. Right away I ordered the twelve-minute video about Bernard's life and yoga practice posted on his website. The video showed Bernard hanging upside down from ropes, bending backward in a yoga chair, and practicing weight-bearing standing poses with the help of a yoga horse, wall ropes, chairs, and blocks.

The poses Bernard demonstrated included all those that older students typically practice in a well-rounded class, such as Standing Forward Bends, Supported Bound-Angle Pose, and Supported Legs Up the Wall Pose. In addition, Bernard demonstrated poses not typically practiced by

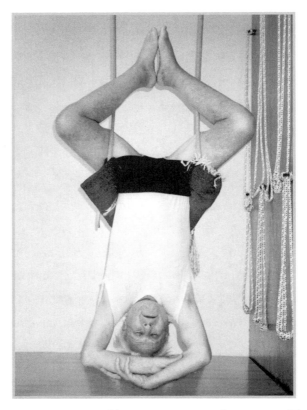

*Bernard Spira practicing Rope **Sirsasana**, at age ninety-two. The benefits of reversing gravity can be experienced at any age.*

*older students, such as hanging upside down in a pelvic sling and hanging from the wall ropes in a Backbend. He also demonstrated a Backbend over a folding chair (**Viparita Dandasana** on a chair) and Supported Shoulderstand with a chair—challenging poses at any age. Watching Bernard's video took my understanding of yoga for seniors to a whole new level!*

Bernard has the good fortune to practice at the B. K. S. Iyengar Yoga Institute of Los Angeles with a team of highly trained teachers who know how to adapt his practice to his body and needs. The institute is set up so students and teachers have convenient access to yoga chairs, blankets, nonskid mats, bolsters, straps, blocks, towels, sandbags, and other props that make yoga more accessible for seniors.

Bernard Spira is an inspiration for everyone who thinks they are too old to go to a yoga class. His level of commitment is exemplary. He pays by the year and attends class almost on a daily basis.

I was so impressed that I decided to interview Bernard about his practice. At the time he was ninety-four years old and still attending classes several times a week. One of his teachers, Marla Apt, told me, "I just had Bernard in class last night—he drove out in the pouring rain—and he continues to inspire me with the challenges he takes on."

I began by asking him the perennial question:

When did you first start practicing yoga?

I started yoga in 1964. I took my first lesson from Indra Devi while on vacation at Rancho La Puerta, a health resort. At that time yoga was a little bit avant-garde. Indra Devi was the first Western woman to travel to India and study with Mr. Iyengar's teacher, T. Krishnamacharya. She was a renowned yoga instructor who taught all over the world.

Indra Devi was one of my first teachers, too, back in the 1970s. I interviewed her in 1995 when she was 94 and still traveling and teaching around the world. She lived to be 102 years old.

Yoga seemed to do me good so I stayed with it for a while. Indra Devi taught me how to stand on my head and all sorts of positions.

After some time passed, however, I dropped it. This was before the days when there were any props.

And then what happened?

At the time I was still working as an aerospace engineer. I was a designer and later became involved in commercial aircraft technology. I began taking aerobics, because it was popular and I wanted to do some strenuous exercise.

A few years later I enrolled in an adult education yoga class with about fifty other students. The teacher was talking about the liver and the intestines and the benefit of yoga for the various organs. I didn't pay much attention to what he said. But, as luck would have it, the teacher of this huge class was none other than Eric Small, who had started practicing Iyengar yoga to help his multiple sclerosis.

Eric was an excellent teacher who motivated me to learn more. He encouraged me to attend the Iyengar Yoga Institute of Los Angeles, where classes were smaller and teachers gave more individual attention and used props. For a time I went from aerobics class straight to yoga.

How old were you when you started classes with Eric Small?

By then I was in my seventies. Eric recalls that I was fairly fit for a man that age but was very stiff.

What was it like going to this style of yoga at a relatively late time of life? What did you think of all the props?

The props are the big help. The teachers adjusting me, showing me how to do the poses properly, were also a big help. The teachers taught me how to position myself so that I could hold the pose longer. They also taught me the poses that work together, that complement each other. This is the whole key to realizing the Iyengar method. If you can't sit down properly with your legs crossed, for example, then the teacher puts blankets under you and then you get the feeling for how to do it.

For many years I slumped over when I sat, and then the teacher came along and put me on two blankets. I now sit straight, and I'm able to stay in the pose and enjoy it. Unless your position is just so—unless it's correct—the pose doesn't work properly, and you don't get the full benefit. It takes a knowledgeable teacher to see what is needed.

Watching you practice, it is evident that your teachers have taught you a lot of special prop setups. How did you learn so much about how to use props?

Learning how to use props was an accumulation of what I learned in class over a period of many years, working with different teachers. When I was eighty-four years old I put in my application to go to India to study at the Ramamani Memorial Institute in Pune, India. I was told I had to wait three years, so I gave up. But my teachers persevered and helped me with the application. When I was eighty-five, I was accepted.

At the time I went to India I was the oldest person at the institute— older even than Mr. Iyengar. When I got there, Marla Apt, a certified Iyengar yoga teacher, told the Iyengars my age, but they were not impressed. To them, age was not an issue.

At that time, Mr. Iyengar was no longer actively involved in teaching, but I took lessons from his children, Geeta and Prashant. From time to time, Iyengar would come to the classes and use me as a model. He once used me to show how Handstand should be done. There were four people assisting under his watchful eye. The way they were supporting me, there was no strain on my wrists or shoulders. It felt very beneficial. With proper support, even older students like me can get the full benefit of turning upside down.

Being in India gave me more confidence to practice yoga a little bit differently. Once I got the knack of it I knew how to adapt myself to any pose. I'm very grateful to Mr. Iyengar and his children.

When I got a little older—late eighties, early nineties—I didn't have the strength to hold the poses in the center of the room, so I started using the yoga horse for stability.

I can feel the affect of the yoga in my body. It feels like I'm giving my body the proper nutrients to stay in shape.

What would you like to tell people about your yoga practice?

If I had not decided to go regularly, on a daily basis, to the Yoga Institute, I would be bending over. I would have problems with scoliosis. When you get older, the spine no longer has that straight position. All the teachers at the Yoga Institute concentrate on helping me to stand up straight and keep in shape.

You cannot do this alone in your home. You can do yoga with a video, but you can't get the maximum benefit! You can only get the maximum benefit by going to a class. Even the teachers attend classes to get the most benefit from yoga.

All of my teachers are interested in yoga therapeutics. They have the ability to conduct the class and take care of me. I'm very fortunate to have teachers who have known me for a long time. I knew most of my teachers when they were beginner students, so they know how to help me practice the pose in a way that is most beneficial.

I want to emphasize again that it is very important to go to class. At home the mind is not fully concentrated. There is nothing like a class! Having a teacher check how you are practicing is as important as going to the doctor for a checkup. There is no place in the medical profession where I can get the therapy I get in a yoga class.

If you just pick up your foot and bring it toward your head that's better than doing nothing. Instead of saying "I'm eighty years old and I can't do it," think that you've had eighty years of experience. Now you're just ripe for this. This is the time to do it. Now! Because what you bring to your practice is your wisdom— the wisdom you've accumulated in your lifetime.

Eric Small, Bernard's yoga teacher, coauthor,
Yoga for Multiple Sclerosis

The body in yoga is used to access the mind. What we are really interested in is to still the chattering of the mind. This is why yoga can be wonderful for seniors. It is not just about glorifying the body, but how to use the body to help quiet the mind.

Karin O'Bannon

Teachers' Comments on
Bernard Spira's Practice

Over the years Bernard has become a sensitive and intelligent yoga practitioner. He can recognize the proper alignment of his muscles, bones, and joints and knows how his breath and inner body should feel in the poses. He can clearly distinguish between good and bad pain and is willing to endure and even welcomes the former. He knows when his posture is not exactly right and when he needs assistance either in the form of a prop or an adjustment.

It is a true pleasure having Bernard at age ninety-four in my classes because he engages fully with the practice. In the course of a single class, I can see the transformative power of yoga working on him.

Marla Apt, Bernard Spira's longtime teacher and faculty member of the Teacher Training Program at Iyengar Yoga Institute of Los Angeles

Bernard (Spira) knows what he can do and what he can't do. He knows how to set up his props and practice to get the most benefit safely. Certainly he requires some help, just like any other student, but here is a man who went to India to study with Iyengar at age eighty-seven. He is a dedicated student. A fabulous yogi!

Leslie Peters, Bernard's yoga teacher

CHAPTER 3

The Greatest Yoga Teachers: Walls and Chairs

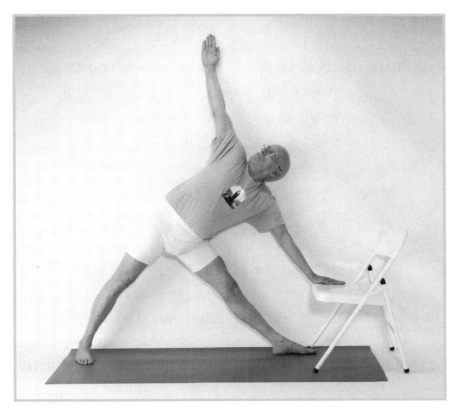

Extended Triangle Pose, **Utthita Trikonasana,** *with the wall and a chair.*

67

*Just as a pebble produces ever widening
concentric ripples on the surface of a still lake,
the positive effects of a yoga practice spread into all aspects
of one's life. As muscle strength, joint flexibility and
neuromuscular coordination improve, one develops
the ability to move with ease and confidence.
This vitally important enhancement of mobility brings
with it independence, self-determination and renewed
interest in life. As exercise tolerance improves, yoga's
salutary effects cascade into a positive, self-perpetuating
cycle, replacing the pernicious negative cycle of
inactivity, deterioration and depression.*

Mary Pullig Schatz, M.D., "Yoga and Aging," *Yoga Journal*

"My Guru, the Wall"

One of the best props for practicing yoga is the wall. Years ago Iyengar wrote a famous article, "My Guru, the Wall," in which he explained how the wall can be your best teacher—in part because it doesn't lie. The support of a wall helps maintain balance and alignment, particularly in standing and inverted poses.

Walls give excellent feedback about our posture both in daily life and when practicing yoga. They remind us to lengthen and align the spine, especially if we are doing many hours of work that tends to round the spine forward. I frequently remind students to stand tall with the backs of their bodies touching a wall or other sturdy structure, for several moments, at least twice a day. The wall provides a convenient reminder not to slouch forward, but to open our chest and lungs and breathe deeply.

People with balance problems gain strength and confidence by practicing standing poses at the wall. A wall provides invaluable support for people who might otherwise be limited to exercise while sitting in a chair or even lying in bed. Walls facilitate weight-bearing postures to strengthen our bones and muscles. The use of walls and other supports also helps us conserve our energy reserves when practicing standing poses. I recommend that you have at least six feet of empty wall space available for practicing standing poses with the back of your body against the wall.

Standing poses can also be practiced by bracing the back foot against a baseboard and holding wall ropes. Examples of this are shown in Chapter 4, "Learning the Ropes." I encourage my older beginners who find it difficult to maintain their balance to practice standing poses at home with the full support of a wall and also with the back foot braced against a wall. Other uses for the wall are described throughout this book.

Innovative Ways to Use Chairs

Chairs can be used in dozens of innovative ways. These ways can be divided into two main categories: first, yoga *with* the assistance of a chair and, second, yoga while actually *seated on* a chair. The latter is popularly known as *Chair Yoga*. You

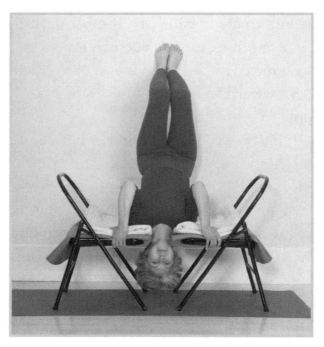

Headstand, **Sirsasana,** *can be practiced with the shoulders supported on two chairs. The head hangs free and there is no pressure on the neck. Inverted poses are empowering and allow us to look at life in a whole new way— upside down!*

will see examples of both these uses of chairs throughout this book.

Many of my older students initially practice standing poses with the help of both a chair and a wall. Safety is another important reason for using walls or chairs, especially for beginners in their seventies and older. When combined with walls and wall ropes, chairs help older people with balance problems to practice yoga without slipping or falling: *The energy that might normally be diverted into struggling to keep your balance can be channeled into practicing the poses correctly and holding them longer.*

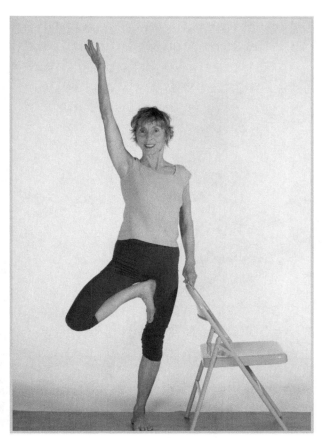

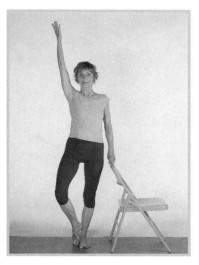

Tree Pose, **Vrksasana,** *begin-ning to balance on one foot, with one hand on a chair.*

Practicing balancing poses like Tree Pose, **Vrksasana,** *improves balance and coordination in daily life.*

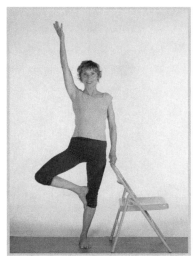

Tree Pose, **Vrksasana,** *bent leg with foot midway up.*

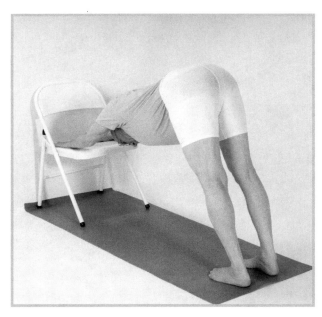

Downward-Facing Dog Pose, **Adho Mukha Svanasana,** *with a Chair.*

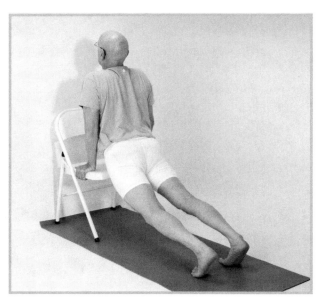

Upward-Facing Dog Pose, **Urdhva Mukha Svanasana,** *with a Chair.*

The Great Yoga Chair

An ordinary metal folding chair with a level seat works well for most chair poses. A sturdy wood, straight-backed chair without sides will also work.

Yoga chairs are made specifically for practicing yoga so there are no rough edges or unpainted metal. They also have extra space between the backrest and the seat so that you can sit backward in the chair, which is convenient for practicing backbends and variations on chair twists. Yoga chairs fold flat for easy storage and have durable, nonmarking feet.

While other armless chairs can also be used for yoga, metal folding chairs are more versatile. They may be used for supported restorative postures and backbends. An inexpensive folding chair can be used in a multitude of ways to stretch and strengthen your body in ways that challenge the most sophisticated gym equipment. You can bend forward, backward, and sideways; do push-ups; relieve backaches and shoulder aches; and go upside down safely with the assistance of this simple piece of furniture. Avoid cushioned or upholstered chairs, since they do not provide a firm, even base of support.

I highly recommend that you invest in a backless, folding yoga chair. All my students who have purchased yoga chairs for home use tell me how much they love their chairs and that they practice more at home. On the other hand, don't let not having a yoga chair be an impediment to your practice! When I teach private lessons in homes with furniture that is too heavy to move around, I sometimes end up demonstrating how to practice yoga with a common metal office chair or outdoor patio chair.

Chair Yoga

I learned many of the chair techniques shown in this book from Eric Small, now in his seventies, who keeps multiple sclerosis in remission by practicing yoga. Eric teaches workshops nationally for people with multiple sclerosis and other problems affecting balance and movement.

In situations where sitting or lying on the floor is not possible or practical, the use of two or more chairs can be very helpful. In unusual situations where students are not able to lower themselves to the floor, even with assistance, I sometimes make a "floor" by using two or more chairs. The surface of the chair becomes like a floor.

Note: *For many older beginners, the single most important part of a yoga class is practicing how to get down and up from the floor with the help of a chair. Chapters 9 and 10 explain how to regain confidence in this essential skill for independent living.*

Ways to Practice Chair Yoga

Following are some innovative ways of practicing with two to four chairs:

Chair 1: The yoga student sits on a sturdy, level, straight-backed chair.

Chair 2: The second chair is about two feet away and directly in front of the student. The student lifts his or her legs one at a time to the level of the seat of the second chair. The student is now sitting in Staff Pose, *Dandasana*.

Chairs 3 and 4: These chairs are placed to the sides of Chair 2. The student can now take his or her feet wide apart, as if sitting in Seated Wide-Angle Pose, *Upavistha Konasana*.

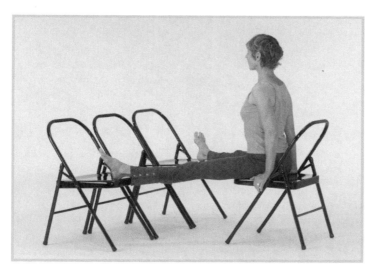

Wide-Angle Pose seated on chairs.

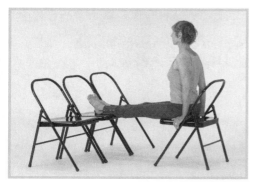
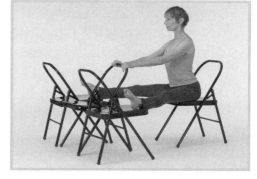

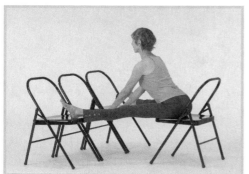
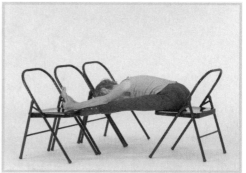

Wide-Angle Pose seated on chairs, bending forward.

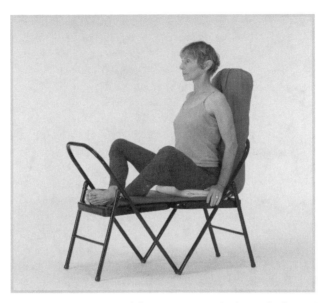

Bound-Angle Pose, soles of feet on second chair, bolster in back.
The support of a bolster helps keep the chest open.

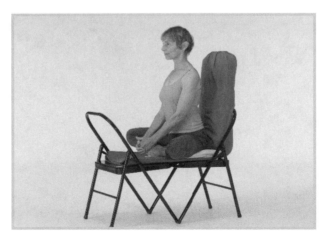

Bound-Angle Pose, holding soles
of the feet, bolster in back.

By moving Chair 2 closer to Chair 1 and padding it with a folded sticky mat, students can bend their knees and bring the soles of their feet together in Bound-Angle Pose, *Baddha Konasana*. While seated, students can stretch their arms up and do shoulder stretches. They can also place their hands on the side edge of the chair seat to help them sit taller.

From here the student can practice many other seated poses, by adjusting the position of the extra chairs. If additional chairs are not available, the student can still practice the chair twist and forward bend shown on pages 78 and 80. Also, small tables or other objects can substitute for a chair.

If the student has difficulty sitting up straight, place a *pranayama* bolster or regular bolster in line with the spine and against the back of the chair. A folded sticky mat on the chair seat helps students feel more comfortable or, in cases where muscles are very weak, from sliding out of the chair. A folded blanket on top of a sticky mat (to keep the blanket from slipping) allows the person to sit forward on the "sit bones," which keeps the spine in an elongated position.

Note: *These instructions can also be helpful for someone who is in a wheelchair. Place the three extra chairs in front of the wheelchair and use them as explained. If circumstances permit, it is psychologically better for the student to get out of the wheelchair and onto the yoga chair.*

For those students who find it impractical to lie on the floor during class, Eric Small makes a bigger "floor" by having the student lie on a surface made out of a row of chairs.

Many examples of how to use chairs to enhance your yoga practice are shown throughout this book. The following are two easy, enjoyable poses to help you get started.

A Rejuvenating Chair Twist

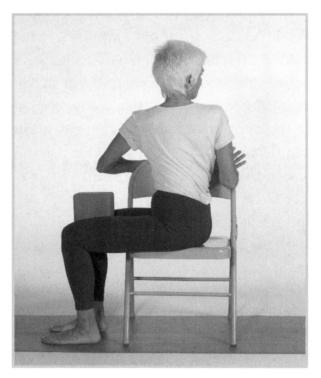

Seated Chair Twist, **Bharadvajasana,** *in a chair.*

- Sit sideways on a chair, with the right thigh/hip against the back of the chair.

- Press your feet firmly into the floor, stretch your shoulders back and down, and lengthen your spine upward. Keep your knees in line with your feet. Bring your hands on the back of the chair. Inhale, lift the spine. Exhale and turn your chest toward the back of the chair.

- Pressing a block between your knees will ensure that you keep the pelvis even and the knees straight. Be sure to keep the knees straight—do not let them splay out—when practicing without a block.

- Continue pressing your feet firmly into the floor as you turn more toward the back of the chair. Pull with the left hand to bring the left side of the body toward the back of the chair. Push with the right hand to turn your right side away from the chair. Keep your upper body stretching upward as you turn as far as you can. Turn your head slowly, and look over your right shoulder.

- Continue twisting for several more breaths; exhale as you come back to the center. Pause for a moment, sitting tall. Move to the opposite side of the chair to repeat the twist on your left side.

Note: *If you are short and your feet do not reach the floor when seated in the chair, place a block, folded yoga mat, or other height under your feet.*

A Relaxing Chair Forward Bend

After the Chair Twist, sit toward the front of the chair. Place your feet wide apart, press firmly into the floor with your feet and stretch your spine upward. Slowly bend forward, keeping the spine elongated and relaxing the back and the head. You can position your arms or place your hands on a stool, bolster, or the floor. This is a relaxing stretch for your back and a

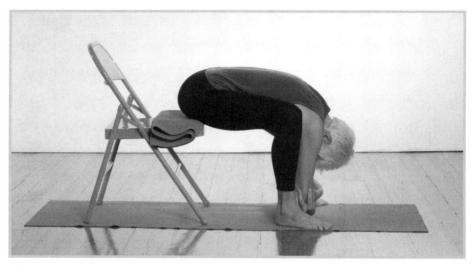

Chair Forward Bend, head down, holding forearms.

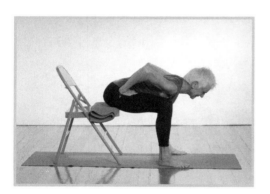

Chair Forward Bend, preparation, hands on hips.

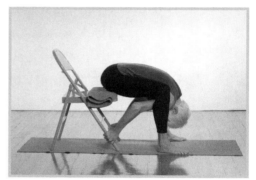

Chair Forward Bend head down, variation, holding front rungs of chair.

gentle, convenient way to improve circulation to the head.

Note: *If bending forward is not relaxing, place the chair near a wall and stretch your hands high up the wall instead of bending forward.*

More ways to use chairs are shown throughout this book. (See Appendix C for information on ordering yoga chairs.)

ELEANOR WILLIAMS

Yoga—a Profoundly Spiritual Experience of the Divine

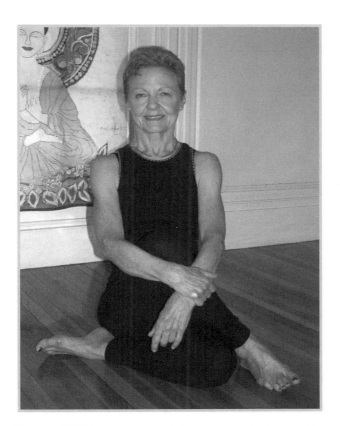

Eleanor Williams began studying yoga in her fifties.

*Physically, yoga is an ideal companion
at this [postmenopausal] stage of life. No matter
what shape your body or mind is in, you can always do
some kind of yoga. Some days you may feel like doing
a vigorous practice; other days your body needs a restorative,
gentle practice; and still other times you may only
have the energy to do deep breathing exercises. No matter
what type of yoga you choose on any particular day,
your body and mind reap profound benefits.*

Patricia Walden, coauthor,
The Women's Book of Yoga and Health

Now in her seventies, Eleanor discovered yoga in her fifties. She is one of the models for The Women's Book of Yoga and Health *and for* Yoga for Healthy Bones, *both coauthored by Linda Sparrowe and Patricia Walden. Eleanor Williams is a yoga teacher in Cambridge, Massachusetts. She studies regularly with Patricia Walden and other Iyengar yoga teachers. Here is Eleanor's yoga story.*

It's widely said that when the student is ready the teacher appears. This is my story.

I was born March 3, 1937, and grew up in the South. I was a child alone and quiet who never ever missed a day of school.

I yearned to be found by God, but never responded to the call from the Altar to surrender to Jesus.

I read Rosicrucian literature all through my teens, and became one of the many who converted to Roman Catholicism.

I had four babies by the time I was twenty-two.

I was not athletic in any way whatsoever. I worked with Moshe Feldenkrais and Ida Rolf, among others, and completed my college degree in time to graduate at the twenty-fifth reunion of my high school class.

At the age of fifty, having graduated from college and married off my children, I needed to find a profession. I passed the Series 7 exams to become a stockbroker. While in the process of being hired to assist a heavy-hitter broker, I began classes at Harvard Divinity School with the idea of becoming a chaplain for teenage girls or for a hospital. I had realized that I was not bold enough to watch people risk their own money, not nice enough to be a psychotherapist, and too rigid to work for the homeless.

While at Harvard Divinity School, I injured my knee. A massage therapist told me, "Your body is quite crooked. It's a wonder you haven't hurt yourself before. Go see Patricia Walden—she'll straighten you out."

It would be a year before I had the fortitude to be straightened out. Patricia advised me that the best thing would be to come to a weekend workshop with Manouso Manos, a senior teacher, so I could really get a sense of what yoga was all about. When I expressed trepidation, Patricia advised: "Just tell the teacher it's your first class."

And so, after fifty-one long years of struggling, my Self and my Soul were reunited.

At the age of fifty-one, having been uncoordinated and afraid of physical activity all of my life, I participated in my first "athletic" event. My first *Savasana* swept over me as a profoundly spiritual experience of the Divine. I was not afraid of the yoga mat, and in *Savasana* I found the God I had so long desired.

I think that yoga was the only hope for me. Not being a natural athlete, coupled with timidity and mild depression, had left me to grow up reading books and cleaning house while waiting for God. The practice and teaching of yoga gave me a spiritual pleasure, an intellectual and athletic adventure, plus a professional involvement and respect I had only seen in others. I settled down and loved myself, my colleagues, my students, and my life. During this time I survived the developing unhappiness of my marriage but was divorced during my sixty-sixth year.

Two years later I realized that I had at most two decades left to live, and I did not want to regret not doing anything that I might be sorry about. I came to the realization that being a *younger older person* is markedly different from being an *older older person*. I took a sabbatical leave from my teaching, which has morphed into a semiretirement.

By the grace of God I can maintain my connection to the Iyengar community and classes with my teacher Patricia Walden. In the meantime, I am learning to play bridge, tennis, and golf and am catching up on my large family and the many wonderful people who have been part of my life's saga.

My primary emotion now is a very deep sense of gratitude and thankfulness. I am profoundly grateful to B. K. S., Geeta, and Prashant Iyengar and to Patricia Walden for this extraordinary gift of yoga.

CHAPTER 4

Learning the Ropes

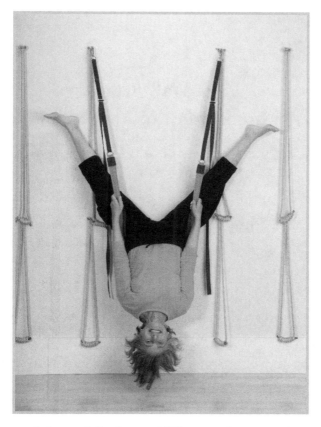

Wall ropes bring out the inner child—even in a seventy-year-old.

Yoga releases the creative potential of Life. . . .
The Light that yoga sheds on Life
is something special.
It is transformative. It does not
just change the way we see things;
it transforms the person who sees.

B. K. S. Iyengar, *Light On Life*

Yoga Wall Ropes:
An Investment in Your Health

Practicing yoga with wall ropes is known as *Yoga Kurunta*. *Kuranti* means "puppet" or "doll made out of wood." When practicing various yoga postures with wall ropes, we become like puppets suspended by ropes. Rope work is both challenging and fun and seems to bring out the ageless inner child in everyone!

B. K. S. Iyengar developed the use of wall ropes. At the Ramamani Memorial Institute in India and in yoga centers and homes around the world, you will find the wall ropes shown in this book and listed in Appendix C, as well as other innovative wall systems with adjustable belts (instead of ropes).

The number and variety of postures and movements that can be done with the ropes is limitless. Once you learn the basics, you can experiment and invent your own ways to use the ropes to explore different yoga poses.

This chapter illustrates the basic poses that can be practiced with wall ropes. The inverted poses should be learned under the guidance of an experienced teacher.

Standing Poses with Wall Ropes

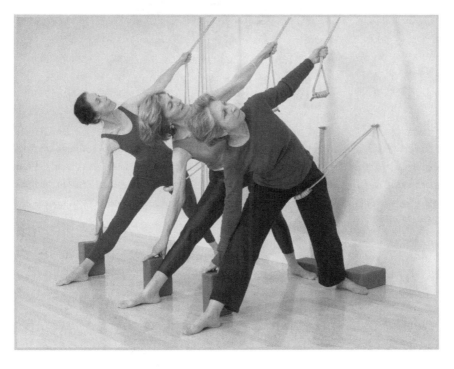

Extended Triangle Pose, **Utthita Trikonasana,** *practiced with the lower rope around the top of back leg, the outer edge of the back foot braced against a block which is placed securely against the wall. The upper hand is holding the upper rope. Practicing standing poses with wall ropes teaches how to extend the spine to the maximum.*

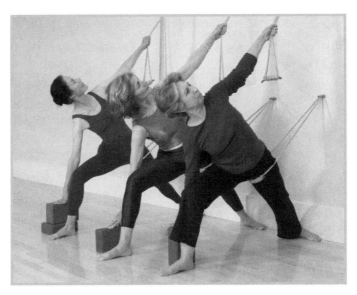

Extended Side-Angle Pose, **Utthita Parsvakonasana,** *practiced with the lower rope around top of the back leg, the edge of the back foot braced against the wall. The upper hand holds the upper rope and the lower hand is on block behind heel.*

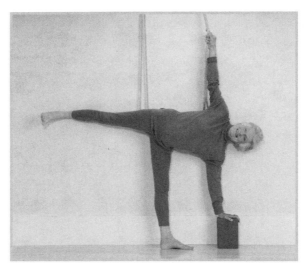

Half-Moon Pose, **Ardha Chandrasana,** *with the back of the body supported by the wall. The upper hand holds the upper rope and the lower hand is on a block or a chair.*

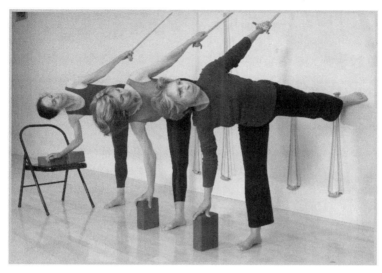

Half-Moon Pose with the back foot pressing into the wall. Upper hand holds the upper rope, the lower forearm or hand is on the chair or a block. Pressing the back foot into the wall helps open the hips and chest and allows the whole body to extend to the maximum.

Deep Stretches with the Upper Ropes

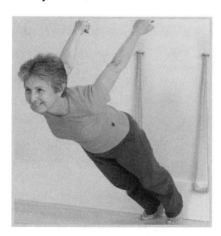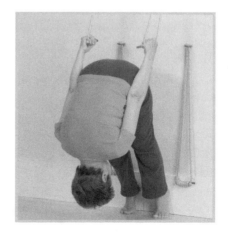

Moving back and forth with the upper ropes from Upward-Facing Dog Pose to a forward bend helps to remove a lifetime of stiffness from the body.

Shoulder Stretches with Wall Ropes

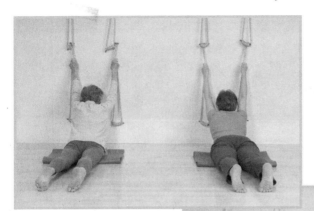

The upper and lower ropes can be used in dozens of ways to extend range of motion in the shoulders.

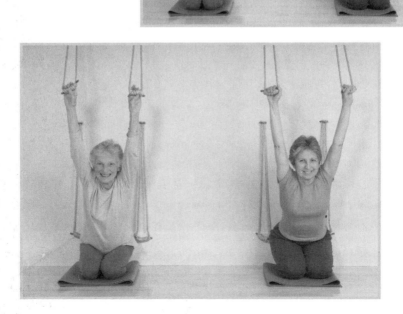

Seated Poses with Wall Ropes

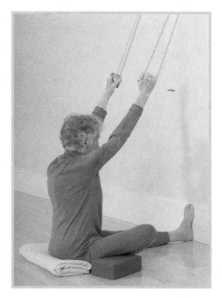

Seated Forward Bend, Head to Knee Pose, **Janusirsasana,** *with upper ropes.*

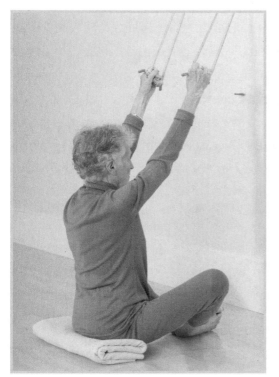

Bound-Angle Pose, **Baddha Konasana,** *can be practiced with both lower and upper ropes to learn to sit straight and elongate the torso when bending forward.*

In my classes and workshops, I use the ropes both to teach the basics of alignment and to help open parts of the body that are difficult to adjust. With the guidance of a skilled teacher, ropes can be used to stretch and strengthen very specific areas of the body.

I also use ropes as therapy for back and neck problems, scoliosis, and joint problems due to arthritis or osteoporosis. Ropes give tremendous support to students who have experienced injuries, surgeries, disabilities, and other medical problems.

One of my seventy-year-old students, Judy, has three pins in one elbow due to an accident, and consequently she cannot completely straighten that arm. Judy can stay only very briefly in poses that require weight bearing in the arms, such as Downward-Facing Dog Pose. For poses that are ordinarily done with straight arms, she usually practices either on her forearms or with a headstand base with her forearms in a tripod on the floor. But when she is suspended in Hanging Downward-Facing Dog Pose, she can stretch to her heart's content, for as long as she likes, and extend both of her arms to their fullest capacity without fear of injuring herself. Perhaps for the same reason, she also delights in hanging upside down in the ropes.

Wall ropes can be used to stretch and strengthen all major muscle groups. They can be used as either support in a pose by providing traction or to help you strengthen an area by providing resistance. They provide support when practicing standing poses, backbends, forward bends, inverted poses, and a wide range of shoulder stretches. Reaching for the upper ropes helps you lengthen your spine and elongate various muscles. When we feel we are too tired to practice, wall ropes help conserve and replenish our energy, which is why they are often used in restorative and therapeutic yoga.

You will not regret investing in a wall rope system. It will take your practice to a whole new level, safely and systematically. Wall ropes are the ideal antidote to the stiffness that tends to settle into the body with the passage of years. Their use helps to counteract feelings of lethargy and to breathe new life into all the systems of the body. Practicing with wall ropes is invigorating and allows us to safely penetrate the deeper levels of poses. See Appendix C for information about the different wall rope systems that are available.

A Note to Older Beginners and Their Teachers: When a ninety-year-old person sits between a set of ropes and is able to reach up and straighten her arms in a way that she may not have done in over a decade, that person feels the same sense of release and exuberance as a younger, advanced practitioner might feel in Upward-Facing Bow Pose. The feeling of bliss that comes when you learn to work with the resistance in your body—not against it—is the same no matter what your chronological age.

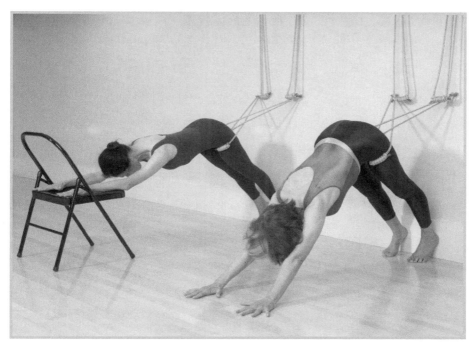

Hanging Downward-Facing Dog Pose is one of the most important poses for improving blood flow to the brain. According to Dr. Raman, it is one of the most useful poses for preventing a stroke.

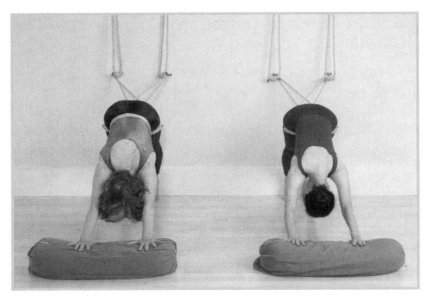

Dog Pose with ropes. The entire weight of the body is taken by the ropes so that there is no strain while holding the pose.

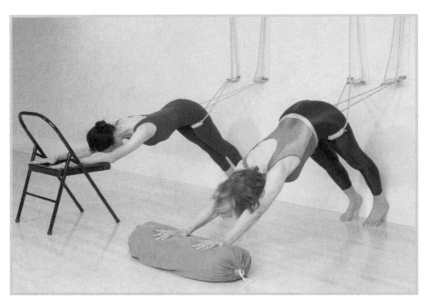

If the stretch at the backs of your legs is too intense, practice Hanging Downward-Facing Dog Pose with your hands on a chair or bolster.

Many of my students have followed my example and now have wall ropes in their homes. It is my hope that this book encourages you to hang ropes at home, and to find a yoga center that has a wall rope system so that you can learn how to get the most benefit from them. When you consider all the equipment that people install in their homes in the last years of life to continue living independently, having someone install a set of ropes will not seem like any trouble or expense.

Benefits of Yoga Ropes

The yoga ropes pull the thighs and pelvis backward, with an effect similar to what happens when a teacher pulls your thighs back with a strap placed at the top of your legs. This allows your spine to fall forward into a delightful, rejuvenating traction. This healing traction relieves back pain and allows you to let go of tension in your whole body, especially the back, neck, and shoulders. The gentle traction of this pose elongates the spinal column, eases back and neck pain, and helps restore an open, youthful posture. I consider this the world's most delicious way to stretch the backs of the legs. It is unequaled for removing tightness in the calves and hamstrings.

In addition, Hanging Downward-Facing Dog Pose and other halfway upside-down poses that place the head below the level of the heart stimulate the endocrine system, including the pituitary gland, which helps regulate hormone levels.

While hanging from a rope is not a substitute for the classic weight-bearing Downward-Facing Dog Pose, practicing in this way allows you to hold the pose much longer, giving the body a rejuvenating stretch without strain. If the backs of your legs are stiff or if you have back problems, place your hands on the seat of a chair (on the back of a chair if you are tall) or a bolster.

Hanging Dog Pose with Ropes

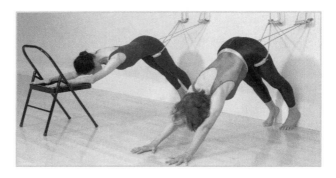

- Stand between the two ropes, with your back to the wall.

- Cross the ropes behind you, and step your left leg into the lower right rope and your right leg into the lower left rope. **Note:** *The ropes should cross behind your bottom.*

- Place the rope knots (handles) into the crease at the very top of your legs between your thighs and torso (also known in yoga as the "hip hinge"). Stand tall with your feet hip-width apart. Step forward until the ropes are taut, being careful not to let them slip down the legs. (If the ropes do slip down, simply press your thighs forward, and bring the ropes back to the top of your legs.)

- Keep the rope taut as you step back toward the wall.

You can adjust the distance between your feet and the wall according to your height and flexibility. Once you get the hang of keeping the ropes taut, hanging with the heels up the wall gives maximum extension to the spine and allows even someone with tight hamstrings to lift his or her pelvis up to create space between the disks.

• Be sure to keep your feet and hands equidistant from the center (midline) and shoulder distance apart, as when practicing Downward-Facing Dog Pose from the floor. Extend your fingertips toward the front of your mat and widely spread apart all ten fingers. Stay in the pose for about a half minute in the beginning, gradually increasing to five minutes or longer.

• You can come out of the pose in several ways. The simplest way is to reverse these directions. Inhale when you come up. Step back toward the wall. Pause for a moment before carefully stepping clear of the ropes.

Caution for Older Students: *Be sure to step back and lean against the wall* before *stepping out of the rope. If you feel dizzy, tell your teacher and hold the pose for less time. Increase the time spent in half and full inverted poses very gradually, with the guidance of an experienced teacher. It is always best for any poses in which the head is below the level of the heart to first practice under the guidance of a knowledgeable teacher.*

Your teacher can show you many wonderful variations and adjustments on these basic ways to practice Hanging Dog Pose.

Downward-Facing Dog Pose
with a Strap

If wall ropes are not available, you can also make a loop out of six to eight feet of soft rope, mountain climbing webbing or other strapping. You will need an open door with two sturdy doorknobs, a chair, and a yoga sticky mat to keep you from slipping.

• Loop the rope around the doorknobs and step into it, placing it at the crease at the top of your thighs.

• Lean forward into the rope, until your weight feels supported, and place your hands on the chair for stability, as illustrated on page 93, Hanging Downward-Facing Dog Pose with a Chair. When you feel secure, and the rope is taut, bring your hands to the floor on your mat, and walk your feet back toward the door. Stay in the pose for at least one minute, breathing deeply without strain, allowing the spine to lengthen. To come out of the pose, walk your hands and feet toward each other, and inhale as you come up.

While nothing beats the convenience and comfort of a set of professional wall ropes, Hanging Dog Pose is practiced in many other ways. When I teach outdoors in nature at yoga retreats, I often make a sturdy loop out of a long yoga strap and hang the strap over a fence post in such a way that the rope doesn't slip.

Hanging Upside Down

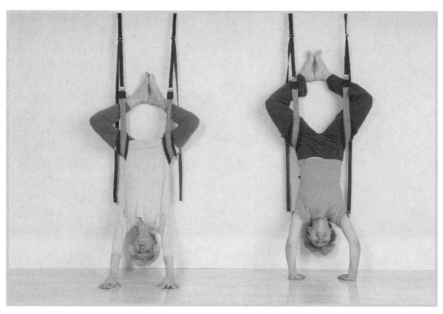

Hanging upside down in a pelvic sling allows people of all ages to reap the rejuvenating benefits of Headstand without straining the neck.

In the world of yoga, hanging completely upside down, as illustrated, is usually referred to as Supported Headstand Hanging from Ropes or Rope *Sirsasana*. (*Sirsasana* is "headstand" in Sanskrit.)

People of all ages, from young children to teenagers to older students like ninety-four-year-old Bernard Spira, enjoy hanging upside down. People at midlife and older, who have the opportunity to try it, have even been known to crave it.

My students often arrive fifteen minutes early so that they can hang upside down before class starts. Even if they've said it a hundred times before, many of them will repeat "Oh! This feels so good!" while they are hanging.

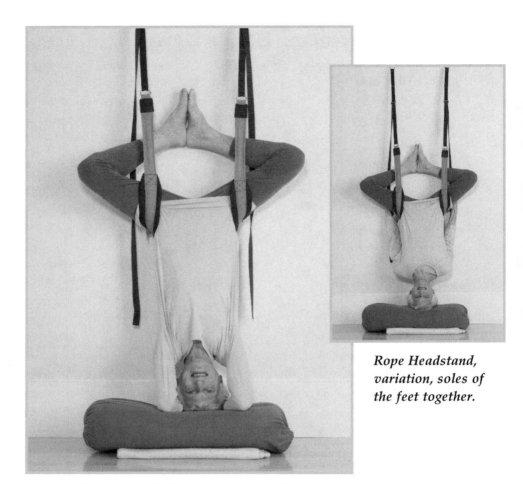

Rope Headstand,
variation, soles of
the feet together.

Supported Headstand, **Sirsasana,** *with wall ropes*
and wide yoga belt or inversion sling.

Dr. Raman points out that in Rope Sirsasana glucose is released from the liver, providing an increase of energy in the brain and a feeling of revitalization. He considers Headstand the single most important asana to prevent a stroke.

In the inverted poses blood supply to the brain, head, and neck is increased with no extra effort on the heart. Better

The Benefits of Hanging Upside Down in Yoga Wall Ropes

There is no strain when we are suspended, as muscular effort is nil. The cranio-facial structures are completely relaxed! The practitioner cannot commit mistakes on the ropes. This helps patients with any medical problem to practice the pose safely. The placement of the ropes is important. We should not use an inversion tilt table. This will make the cerebral flow heavy and uncomfortable.

Imagine a geriatric patient with Cervical Spondylosis practicing Headstand on the floor without proper medical guidance. The ropes provide confidence and protect such patients. Medically, when we want to achieve benefits faster and work against time, the ropes are of great help. Unless we have a fear of suspension, the ropes are very helpful. We can overcome such phobias if we attempt the pose. Later we will realize that the fear was irrational. The main difference between practicing Headstand independently and on the ropes is that, on the ropes, the thoracic and abdominal organs are stretched and flattened intensely.

Independent practice of Headstand is a "psychological pose" as we need confidence for the balance. Headstand on the ropes is a ventilator of the abdominal and thoracic organs—an effect not available with Headstand done independently. The blood circulates better in the abdominal and thoracic organs.

Krishna Raman, M.D.,
Yoga and Medical Science

circulation improves the functioning not only of the brain but of the endocrine glands located in the head and neck—the pituitary gland, the hypothalamus, the pineal and thyroid gland—and of the sense organs in the head.

In all the inverted poses, blood supply to the brain, head, and neck is improved with no extra effort required of the heart. Better circulation improves functioning not only of the brain but also the endocrine glands in the head and neck.

In Supported Headstand, the pituitary and the adrenal glands receive the benefit of improved oxygenation, which gives the mind and body a peaceful and energetic feeling. The entire weight of the body is taken by the rope so there is no strain. In this way the benefits of being inverted—of reversing gravity—can be obtained at any age.

Reversing gravity is especially beneficial for the internal organs. As we age, our organs grow fatigued, lose suppleness and function less efficiently. The loss of suppleness is due in part to the constant downward pull of gravity on all the soft tissues of the body. Inverting the body not only rests the internal organs from gravity's pull but also stretches and tones them. Such tissues perform better and age with greater vitality.

The unique combination of stretching and traction produced by hanging upside down also offers relief for many types of back and neck pain. Stretching helps to relieve muscle tension and spasm, while gravity pulls the spine into gentle traction, opening the spaces between the vertebrae. The opening relieves pain caused by pressure on spinal nerves and disks.

After the practice of inverted poses, you feel replenished and rejuvenated. You feel good from the inside out! As we grow older, the feeling of increased energy and revitalization in the body and brain that occurs after practicing inversions cannot be overemphasized.

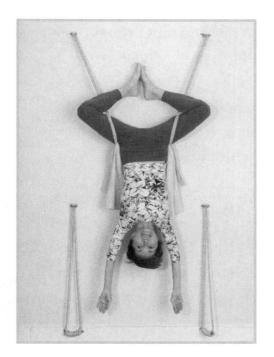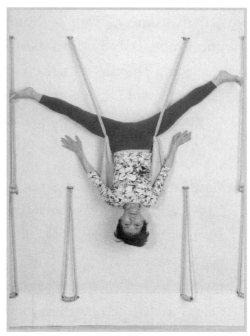

Hanging upside down, soles of the feet together and feet wide apart, has the added benefit of stretching the inner thigh muscles. Extending the arms gives a wonderful stretch to the neck, back, chest, and shoulder muscles.

Effects of Inversions on Internal Organs

Reversing gravity is beneficial to our internal organs. As we age, our organs lose their suppleness, grow fatigued, and function less efficiently. Loss of suppleness results, in part, from gravity's continual downward pull on all the soft tissues of the body, including our internal organs. Inverting the body helps preserve the resilience of our soft tissues by reversing the direction in which gravity pulls them. The reversal not only rests our organs from gravity's pull but stretches and tones them; rested and toned, they perform better and age more vitally.

Placing the soles of the feet together in Bound-Angle Pose (*Baddha Konasana*) has the added benefit of stretching the inner thigh muscles. Extending the arms gives a wonderful stretch to the neck, back, chest, and shoulder muscles.

Caution: *While halfway upside-down postures such as Hanging Dog Pose are safe for almost everyone, turning the body completely upside down may not be appropriate for some people. Complete inversions are not recommended for people with hiatal hernias, eye pressure, or retinal problems. Check with your teacher if you have hypertension or if you are using blood thinners or other medications.*

For people new to practicing inversions, it is wise to practice halfway upside-down poses such as Downward-Facing Dog Pose (either hanging from the rope or from the floor) before turning your body completely upside down. Gradually increase the length of time you stay inverted. Rest by bending your knees to the floor. Separate your knees about hip-width apart, big toes touching. Lower your bottom back toward your heels as you fold your torso onto your thighs and lay your forehead on the floor or a folded blanket (Child's Pose). Rest in Child's Pose for at least one minute.

Note: *Yoga wall rope systems and inversion slings come with instructional booklets, but it is best to have a knowledgeable teacher present to assist you with proper technique. All inverted poses should be learned under the guidance of an experienced teacher.*

Sulochana D. Telang, M.D., on Elderly Persons in Rope *Sirsasana*

An elderly man of 75 years was in Rope *Sirsasana*. After a little while, he developed a pinkish blue hue of congestion over his face and neck, and looked distressed. I thought that his cerebral circulation was in danger. So I pointed this out to Guruji. He promptly gave a bolster and a pillow underneath the patient's hanging head to support it. Within 3 to 5 seconds the congestion of head and face disappeared, and the skin assumed a healthy pink color and a peaceful look.

I tried to analyze this phenomenon in the light of medical knowledge. In a normal young person the blood pressure receptors in the carotid arteries (blood vessels to the head and neck) get stimulated when the pressure becomes high as in inverted Asana poses. The stimulation of these receptors causes constriction of the cerebral arterioles. This stops the high-pressure blood flow from reaching the brain capillaries. If it does not do so the capillaries can rupture causing brain hemorrhage. Thus this pressure receptor response is a protective mechanism for the brain circulation. In this elderly person of 75 years of age, this protective pressure receptor nervous mechanism had probably failed because of his advanced age.

Sulochana D. Telang, M.D.,
Understanding Yoga Through Body Knowledge

CARIN SEEBOLD

At Sixty-Something, We're Just Getting Started

"You'll never stick with this!" I remember so clearly these words spoken by a relative when I first began studying yoga.

I was fifty-three years old when I started taking yoga classes. Now here I am, over sixty, still taking classes twice a week, practicing at home as often as I can, and teaching one day a week. So, while this relative thought she knew me, she didn't realize how yoga can become a serious habit that permeates your entire being.

Looking back, I see numerous positive effects of yoga on my life. These include my easy transition through menopause, my exploratory journeys into alternative health and nutrition, and my gradual change of attitude from outward materialism to inward spirituality. I believe wisdom comes with age, as does introspection, but yoga has definitely influenced my path in this direction.

Another obvious benefit of a regular yoga practice for men and women over sixty is the physical aspect. My only real physical complaint at this age is arthritis in my fingers. I do not take any medications for this and have never felt it impeded my lifestyle. I attribute this to my yoga practice. I have practiced specific finger exercises since I first read about them in Suza's book *The New Yoga for People Over 50*.

Yoga enhances both stamina and strength. It keeps muscles long and lean. It builds bone strength and teaches balance. It may not generate actual weight loss, but it certainly allows one to maintain a healthy weight.

Yoga can work just as well for the overweight or physically challenged as it can for anyone else. There are so many different types of yoga available; there is something that can work for everyone. While my background is based on Iyengar yoga, I have explored other branches of hatha yoga, including Kundalini, which has given me a more rounded approach.

A natural progression for me has been teaching students who live in my retirement community. I am lucky enough to have a small room (ten by ten) that I have devoted to my yoga practice. I have a wood floor, a yoga "wall," and plenty of props.

My students are in their sixties to mid-seventies. My goal is to introduce them to yoga by teaching them the basics. Then, when and if they choose, they can move on to a yoga center for more classes. It gives me such joy and warmth to be able to share my love of yoga with my friends and neighbors.

Yoga is a perfect adjunct to continuing senior health. It can be done anywhere, anytime, and without machinery or equipment, although props do enhance practice. It invites meditation, which has proven so helpful to coping with many diseases. It always includes a relaxation period to nurture and encourage complete letting go.

Even in retirement, people are sometimes overly busy and need to relax. In yoga, there is no competition. Everyone can progress at their own pace. It is one of the few activities that can be done well into old age (and what is old age these days?). Instead of wearing out body parts, it builds them up.

If you haven't already tried yoga, expand your horizons and enroll in a local beginner class. If you're already an aficionado, keep up the good work. You and I will be doing yoga at seventy, eighty, and ninety, just like the models in this book. At sixty-something, we're just getting started!

FELICE RHIANNON

A Refreshed New Way of Being

*F*elice is an "over sixty" yoga teacher who specializes in working with midlife and older students.

*T*he comparing mind is a dangerous thing.
By leaving the present moment—whether at thirty or at sixty—
we abandon the most precious awareness we have.
Classical yoga texts teach us that the third and fourth stages
of life are devoted to developing wisdom and insight into life's
meaning. Pranayama and meditation are the primary practices
suggested for these phases, although maintaining health,
strength, and flexibility with asana is also vital.
The blessings of these stages far surpass the aches and pains.
They are our legacy to those who follow. By honoring
the wisdom and experience of elders, our world will not
only change from its current youth-driven frenzy but
will also become a more peaceful place to live.

Felice Rhiannon, *Yoga Journal*

At the age of fifty-two, I was confined to my bed with chronic illness for a year. It was the worst year of my life. On a "good" day I could wash dishes. On a bad day I had to crawl on hands and knees to the bathroom. I was under treatment but still feeling awful.

I became deeply depressed, not only as a side effect of the illness itself but at my inability to live the life I so deeply wanted. I had just completed my training to be a yoga teacher, and instead of teaching I was flat on my back! I had all but given up hope to ever teach again.

One day it occurred to me that I might make use of my training by practicing yoga in bed. And, having nothing else to do, I made an attempt. Energy, albeit just a little, began to flow through me in a way so familiar and so deeply missed. I began to experiment as I gained some strength and hope.

Over the next several months I progressed from bed to floor; floor to chair; and, finally, to standing on my own two feet, practicing modified yoga postures that I designed to meet my abilities and needs. I was so excited! By then I was thoroughly convinced of the therapeutic value of yoga. Not only was my body stronger, but my mental and emotional states were more balanced, and my stress level had dropped dramatically.

Living a full, rewarding life with an open mind and a mobile body is the gift of yoga. Because I feel more alive than I have in years, enjoying a new-found sense of peace and contentment, I had to share this gift. As soon as my health improved enough, I enrolled in the therapeutic yoga training course and am now a fully certified professional yoga therapist.

"I can't practice yoga. I'm not flexible!" This common misconception prevents many people in their middle and senior years from enjoying the life-enhancing benefits of a yoga practice. Nothing could be further from the truth.

Yoga offers—to every man and woman in their middle years and beyond—a refreshed, new way of being, in body, mind, heart, and spirit, regardless of age or physical capacity. The adaptable, individualized techniques of yoga let you enjoy its benefits no matter what your current age or physical condition.

One of yoga's premier qualities is its ability to bring deep relaxation to the body and mind, ushering in calm and tranquility. By relieving stress, yoga helps remove perhaps the most destructive factor in the aging process. So many contemporary illnesses are stress related. Yoga can help to reduce or eliminate many of the conditions that arise in the middle years, including high blood pressure, heart disease, migraines, irritable bowel syndrome, and ulcers, arthritis, and poor posture.

So you still think you can't practice yoga? Yes, you can! And you can enjoy a great many more years of vibrant well-being.

CHAPTER 5

Beautiful Bones
for Life

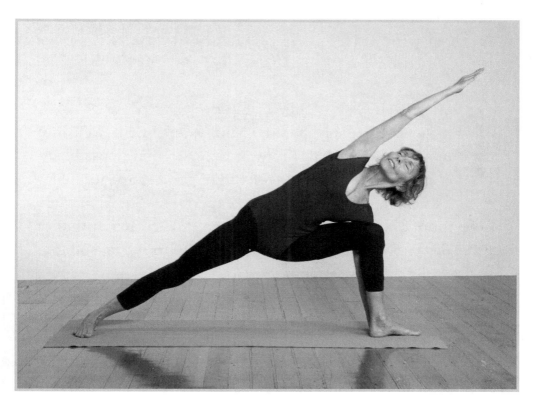

Extended Side-Angle Pose, **Utthita Parsvakonasana.** *Yoga's beautiful stand-ing poses create strong bones, flexible joints, youthful posture, and better balance in daily life.*

The ancient Indian philosophy of yoga offers a much-needed unified and holistic approach to bone health. This approach has nothing to do with clinical trials or changing scientific opinions. Rather the yoga perspective has everything to do with alignment, balance, harmony, and a life lived in accordance with natural laws.

Susan E. Brown, Ph.D., C.C.N.,
Director of the Osteoporosis Education Project, from
the foreword to *Yoga for Healthy Bones*

I f you want to stay healthy and independent well into your real old age, start now to do everything possible to keep the bones of your skeleton in good shape for a lifetime. According to bone health expert Dr. Susan Brown, Director of the Osteoporosis Education Project, and author of *Better Bones, Better Bodies*, it is *never* too late to begin building and rebuilding bone strength.

Osteoporosis affects approximately 44 million people and leads to 1.5 million fractures per year, mostly in the hip, spine, and wrist. The annual cost of treatment is estimated at $17 billion, and it is rapidly increasing, reminding us of the wisdom that "Prevention is cheaper than cure."

Both men and women get osteoporosis. One in two women and one in four men over age fifty will suffer a vertebral (spinal) fracture. *Osteoporosis*, which means "porous bones," is a condition of skeletal fragility resulting in bones that break easily. Myriad causes are responsible for low bone density and decreased bone strength. A combination of genetic, environmental, dietary, hormonal, age-related, and lifestyle factors all contribute to this condition.

Yoga's holistic approach to a strong, aligned skeletal structure is an intelligent alternative to the fragmented, short-sighted approaches that recommend swallowing a weekly or monthly pill to prevent our bones from falling apart.

Maybe you're not terribly worried
about your bones, joints, and muscles right now,
but they're hugely important to the way we age, if for
no other reason than this: Having Lance Armstrong's
heart or Albert Einstein's brain doesn't mean a darn
thing if you can't lift yourself off the toilet.

Mehmet Oz, M.D., and **Michael Roizen, M.D.,**
You: The Owner's Manual

Weight-Bearing Exercise that Doesn't Wear You Out

Exercise makes bones and muscles stronger and prevents bone loss. Exercise also helps us to stay active and mobile as we grow older. Bone is living tissue that responds to exercise by becoming stronger, just as muscles do. When you are inactive, your bones do not receive any messages that they need to stay strong and dense. Particularly as we grow older, this contributes to lower bone mass and density.

If you are already diagnosed with osteoporosis (decreased bone mineral density, resulting in porous bones) or osteopenia (low bone mineral density, a precursor to osteoporosis), you may feel you face a classic Catch-22 position: You are advised to do weight-bearing impact exercises that force you to work against gravity and bear weight on your bones, joints, and muscles. Such exercise is needed to stimulate cells that build bone but actually can result in joint destruction and bone fractures.

Weight-bearing exercise stimulates a mini electrical current in your skeleton that draws strengthening minerals right into the bone matrix. A well-rounded yoga practice includes weight-bearing postures and takes your body through its full range of motion; lengthens your spine; opens your posture; and stretches and strengthens your muscles in a balanced way, which reduces wear and tear on your joints.

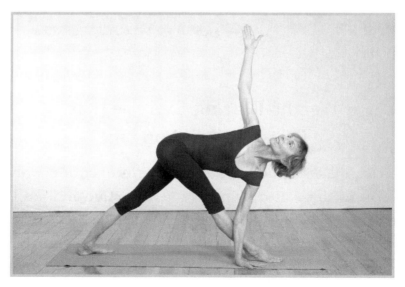

Revolved Triangle Pose, **Parivritta Trikonasana,** *a weight-bearing pose that won't wear you out!*

The challenge as we grow older is to exercise in a way that does not contribute to bone fractures or have a negative effect on our joints. The usual forms of weight-bearing high-impact exercise, such as jogging and various other sports, are known to stimulate the cells that build bone. Unfortunately, with the passage of time, such forms of movement often contribute to joint destruction that can result in hip and knee replacements (see Chapter 7).

Recent studies report that yoga improves the actual congruence of joints, undoing (reversing) the wear and tear that is responsible for osteoarthritis (see Chapter 6). Nonimpact, nonweight-bearing exercise, such as swimming, won't wear out your joints, but it won't strengthen your bones either. The good news is that a balanced yoga practice can give you all the positive benefits of weight-bearing exercise without negative wear and tear on the joints!

Homeostasis: A Stable Internal Environment

Our amazing human bodies have numerous backup systems working day and night to keep us stable and balanced; this is known as *homeostasis*.

The ability to maintain a stable internal environment, even under less than desirable conditions, allows the body to keep functioning for as long as it does. For our bones, homeostasis regulates the body's use of calcium.

The teeth and skeleton are particularly good storehouses for calcium, and the body needs a great deal of calcium, around the clock, to maintain vital functions. Calcium is needed not

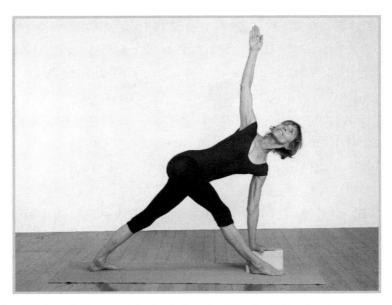

Revolved Triangle Pose with the help of a block. Older beginners can practice this pose with their bottom hand on a chair.

just for strong bones and teeth, but also for clotting the blood, transmitting nerve impulses, ensuring muscle movement and growth, regulating the heart's rhythm, and stabilizing the nervous system.

Ninety-nine percent of the body's calcium is stored in the skeleton. The remaining 1 percent must take care of all of calcium's other vital functions in the soft tissues of the body. If necessary, to meet this urgent demand, calcium is pulled from our bones. If our diet is deficient in replenishing the calcium that is used, our bones can lose up to one-third of their calcium without immediate detriment to our system.

Over time, however, a continuing loss causes the bones to become soft and porous and may cause osteoporosis, osteopenia, and related degenerative disorders, including back and disk problems, bone fractures, and pyorrhea (loss of bone surrounding the teeth). From this perspective, as Susan Brown points out, osteoporosis is really the body's intelligent action in response to long-term imbalances and stresses.

Rethinking Bone Density

Researchers have measured the bone density of people with broken bones and found that 25 percent had osteoporosis, 25 percent had high bone density and 50 percent had normal bone density. People with high bone density broke their hips as frequently as those with osteoporosis did!

Bone density readings do one thing and one thing only: They read bone density. They don't measure bone strength or quality, and these factors determine if bone is more likely to fracture. Bone density is measured as "mineral content per measured area unit"—or the amount of bony material in a specific space. But as Susan Love, M.D., points out in *Dr. Susan Love's Hormone Book,* "We don't in reality know what 'normal' bone density should be."

Low bone density is not necessarily a sign of brittle bone. If bone quality is good, you can actually lose 25 percent or more of your bone mass and still resist fractures. In fact, it's normal to lose a bit of bone as you get older, but that doesn't mean your bones must get brittle. Women who have small bones may have low bone density because their bones have never been very dense—not because they have true osteoporosis.

To learn more about bone testing and the different tests available to assess the current state of your bones, visit www.betterbones.com.

To Avoid Brittle Bones, Eliminate All Risk Factors

*Our bones are dynamic,
constantly changing tissues, connected
minute-by-minute to our entire mind-body system.
Every morsel we eat, every move we make, and
every thought we have affects our bones.*

Susan E. Brown, Ph.D., C.C.N.
Director of the Osteoporosis Education Project, from
the foreword to *Yoga for Healthy Bones*

Anything that inhibits the body's ability to absorb calcium contributes to the likelihood of osteoporosis. Sugar is by far the main dietary culprit. Researchers have found that ingesting sugar increases the rate at which we excrete calcium. Unfortunately, taking extra supplemental calcium to combat this depletion, if it is not in the proper ratio to other minerals, can cause numerous other health problems, including kidney stones, bone spurs, arthritis, and hardening of the arteries.

Many other substances in the modern diet affect the body's ability to absorb calcium. Ingestion of large quantities of caffeine leads to calcium and other nutrient loss through the urine. Consumption of phosphoric acid in soft drinks causes calcium to be pulled from bones. Alcohol, smoking, aluminum from cookware and other sources, softened water and water from other sources, excess sodium from salt and many common medications, anti-inflammatory drugs, and steroids also interfere with calcium availability.

Increasing your exposure to sunlight will ensure you obtain adequate doses of vitamin D, an essential bone-building vitamin. The vitamin D produced under your skin in sunny weather is stored by your body for use during the winter.

Soft Drinks and Osteoporosis

All soft drinks are made with a solution of phosphoric acid. This is, in part, what gives them their kick. Phosphorous is a very active element, having the ability to combine with calcium. Most people have a poor calcium intake. The phosphorus then pulls the calcium from their storage warehouse—that is, their teeth and bones. The result is osteoporosis—that is, loss of density of bones, back and disc trouble, pyorrhea and, of course, decayed teeth. The sugar, three to six teaspoons per six ounces of soft drink, of course, multiplies the problem.

George E. Meinig, D.D.S., FACD, "New"trition

Yoga for a Lifetime of Better Bone Health

Yoga is the ideal exercise prescription for prevention of osteoporosis, for those already at risk, and for bone regeneration. The 206 bones in the human body are living, breathing, changing tissue that requires a steady supply of blood and nutrients and a flow of energy or *prana*. Yoga postures, besides providing a superior form of weight-bearing exercise that stimulates bones to retain calcium, also help stimulate and distribute the flow of

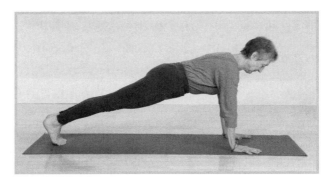

Plank Pose, also known as a yoga push-up, stimulates the bones to retain calcium, and strengthens the bones in the shoulders, wrists, elbows, as well as the legs, knees, and ankles.

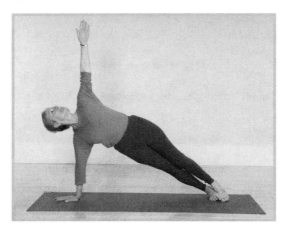

Plank Pose with one arm up, **Vasisthasana I.**

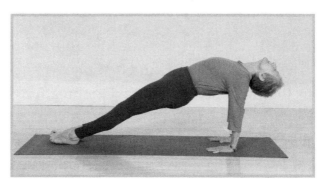

Reverse Plank Pose, for more experienced students.

synovial fluid, which lubricates the joints between the bones. Jogging, dancing, weight lifting, racquet sports, and other forms of exercise, while strengthening bones, may cause further imbalance in the muscular system. Conversely, yoga postures balance the muscular system while bones are strengthened. When the muscular system is balanced, the skeletal system is brought back into alignment, reducing the risk of wear-and-tear conditions such as osteoarthritis.

Ten Reasons Why Yoga Builds Better Bone Strength at Any Age

1. Yoga is one of the few exercise systems in which weight is borne through the entire body. In weight-bearing standing poses, inverted poses, active backbends, and various arm balances, weight is systematically applied to the bones in the hands, wrists, arms, upper body, neck and head, feet, and large bones of the legs and hips.

2. Because yoga postures are learned gradually, the weight applied to the bones increases safely and incrementally, as the student becomes stronger and can hold postures for longer periods.

3. While building strength, yoga poses simultaneously promote mobility in the hips and shoulders, remove stiffness in the joints, and bring flexibility to the whole body.

4. Standing poses and other poses that require one to strongly engage the bones and muscles of the legs affect the pelvis and spine. This increases circulation and benefits the health of the whole body.

5. Yoga prevents and can even reverse the most visible and obvious symptom of osteoporosis and aging: the rounding of the spine. Yoga poses encourage concavity of the spine, rather than a convex humped shape.

6. Weight bearing through the arms and upper spine in poses such as Downward-Facing Dog and the weight-bearing inversions keep the upper spine strong. Yoga's upper-body weight-bearing poses are particularly beneficial in preventing the hairline fractures in the vertebrae that result in the upper-back curvature common in older people.

7. While other weight-bearing exercises tighten the body and wear out the joints, yoga increases flexibility and "lubricates" the joints by giving them an internal massage.

8. Seated postures help keep our hip joints healthy as they require a wide range of movements that increase mobility.

9. Yoga postures also have a balancing effect on the endocrine glands, which contributes to the formation of strong, healthy bones. Restorative yoga poses replenish the adrenal glands, thus reducing stress levels and inhibiting excess calcium secretion. Supported backbends—which can be as mild as restorative poses, such as lying over a bolster, or more intense, such as using a chair as support—promote deep relaxation and restore the health of the endocrine system.

10. Yoga improves balance and coordination, helping to prevent falls. Agility and flexibility derived from a range of movement help us to maintain our balance and avoid falls.

*Sitting twists "squeeze and soak" the
intervertebral disks, the (relatively) round, spongy
pads that separate the spinal vertebrae; the principle is
much like squeezing and soaking a sponge. The twisting
movement itself squeezes the disk, wringing out all
the "dirty water"; then when you release the twist,
"clean water"—spinal fluids and blood—is soaked up.
This keeps the disks supple well into old age.*

Richard Rosen, *Yoga for 50+*

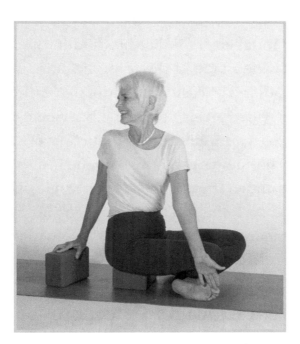

Seated-Twist in Cross-Legged Pose, Easy Pose, **Sukhasana,** *seated on a block, back hand on a block. Twists increase flexibility of the spine and may help prevent height loss.*

Yoga and Preventing Height Loss

Decreased height is not always the result of bone loss. Years of poor posture and lack of stretching can also make us shorter than we once were. Some height loss results from the shrinking of spaces between vertebral disks, even when bone density is good. Yoga helps keep the space between the vertebrae open, plump, and supple. Many of my older students report that they have regained lost height. Similarly, when students who have experienced some height loss stand very tall and strong, the height loss is not noticeable.

Reducing Stress Helps Keep Your Bones Healthy

A growing number of studies are finding that stress contributes to a wide range of diseases, including osteoporosis. Cortisol and other corticosteroid hormones, if they remain in the body at elevated levels due to the body being in a state of continual stress, can inhibit the production of estrogen and progesterone, hormones essential for bone health. In addition, when we are under stress, our blood becomes slightly more acidic, which, over time, removes calcium from the bones. When we are more relaxed, our blood becomes more alkaline, and we don't lose as much calcium.

Safe Yoga for Osteoporosis

If you've been diagnosed with osteoporosis or if you have lost a significant amount of bone mineral density, be sure to inform your teacher about your condition before attending classes. Study with a teacher who understands osteoporosis and who can give you appropriate guidance either privately or within a class setting.

Keep in mind that it is possible to not even be aware that you've broken any bones. If you've lost two or more inches in height, you have probably already experienced vertebral fractures.

I teach students of all ages how to move with maximum awareness, as well as how to move from their "hip hinge" with the upper body in one unit. As other teachers who are concerned about osteoporosis have pointed out, "Hinge at the hips" is the general rule. Unfortunately, stiff beginning students have a difficult time actually doing this. If the hamstring muscles at the backs of the thighs are tight, it is difficult to bend forward without rounding, and consequently compressing, the back—especially in the thoracic spine (the midback), which is the area most at risk for fracture.

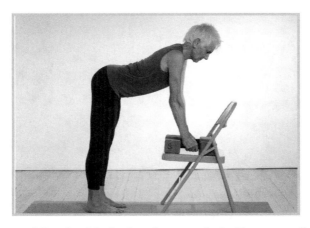

Standing Forward Bend with the hands on a chair. Props can help you bend forward safely from your hip joint without straining your lower back.

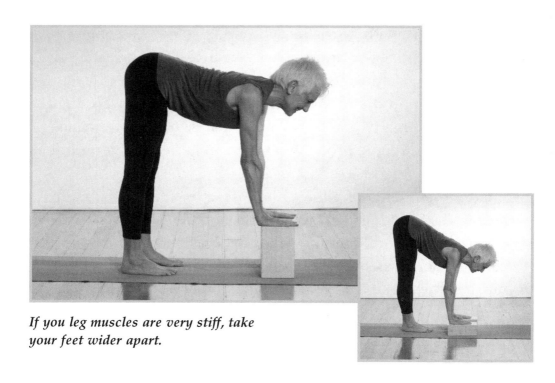

If you leg muscles are very stiff, take your feet wider apart.

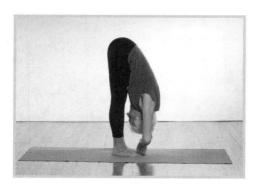

The classic Standing Forward Bend Pose, **Uttanasana.** *Note how the upper body bends forward in one unit, from the hip hinge.* **Never** *bounce or strain to touch the floor.*

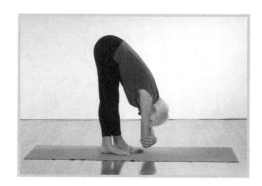

Relaxing variation, holding the elbows.

READER/CUSTOMER CARE SURVEY

We care about your opinions! Please take a moment to fill out our online Reader Survey at **http://survey.hcibooks.com**.

As a **"THANK YOU"** you will receive a **VALUABLE INSTANT COUPON** towards future book purchases as well as a **SPECIAL GIFT** available only online! Or, you may mail this card back to us and we will send you a copy of our exciting catalog with your valuable coupon inside.

(PLEASE PRINT IN ALL CAPS)

First Name _____ MI. _____ Last Name _____

Address _____

State _____ Zip _____ Email _____ City _____

1. Gender
- ❑ Female
- ❑ Male

2. Age
- ❑ 8 or younger
- ❑ 9-12
- ❑ 13-16
- ❑ 17-20
- ❑ 21-30
- ❑ 31+

3. Did you receive this book as a gift?
- ❑ Yes
- ❑ No

4. Annual Household Income
- ❑ under $25,000
- ❑ $25,000 - $34,999
- ❑ $35,000 - $49,999
- ❑ $50,000 - $74,999
- ❑ over $75,000

5. What are the ages of the children living in your house?
- ❑ 0 - 14
- ❑ 15+

6. Marital Status
- ❑ Single
- ❑ Married
- ❑ Divorced
- ❑ Widowed

7. How did you find out about the book?
(please choose one)
- ❑ Recommendation
- ❑ Store Display
- ❑ Online
- ❑ Catalog/Mailing
- ❑ Interview/Review

8. Where do you usually buy books?
(please choose one)
- ❑ Bookstore
- ❑ Online
- ❑ Book Club/Mail Order
- ❑ Price Club (Sam's Club, Costco's, etc.)
- ❑ Retail Store (Target, Wal-Mart, etc.)

9. What subject do you enjoy reading about the most?
(please choose one)
- ❑ Parenting/Family
- ❑ Relationships
- ❑ Recovery/Addictions
- ❑ Health/Nutrition
- ❑ Christianity
- ❑ Spirituality/Inspiration
- ❑ Business Self-help
- ❑ Women's Issues
- ❑ Sports

10. What attracts you most to a book?
(please choose one)
- ❑ Title
- ❑ Cover Design
- ❑ Author
- ❑ Content

FOLD HERE

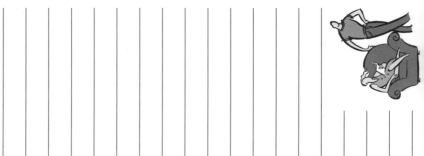

Comments

Yoga for Osteoporosis: Guidelines and Cautions

1. **Avoid high-impact exercise and sudden jerking, rapid movements.** High-impact exercise is hard on joints and not recommended for people who already have osteoporosis; balance problems; or knee, ankle, or back problems. High-impact exercise that involves bouncing while stretching, or rapid stretching with poor body alignment, may cause crush fractures of weakened vertebrae and exacerbate existing problems due to osteoporosis and poor posture.

2. **Avoid activities that reinforce a rounding of the upper (thoracic) spine (kyphosis) or hunched, collapsed positions that exacerbate poor posture.** All activities in which the upper body is hunched can intensify the forces that result in vertebral crush fractures. This includes hunching while attempting to touch your toes in a standing or seated forward bend. It is especially important for menopausal women at risk for osteoporotic fractures to practice yoga's seated poses with adequate props.

3. **Avoid hyperextension of the neck. Do not tilt your head way back.** This action can potentially compress the vertebral arteries and interrupt blood flow to the brain, possibly causing fainting or even a stroke. When lying down, place adequate support under your head to keep your forehead level or slightly higher than your chin. A forward-head position and rounded upper back usually precede the vertebral wedge fractures that result in dowager's hump.

4. **Avoid poses that bear weight directly on the neck. Weak, porous vertebrae are vulnerable to injury.** People at high risk for osteoporosis should practice weight-bearing inverted poses such as Headstand and Shoulderstand only under the guidance of an experienced instructor. If you are new to yoga and have osteoporosis, Headstand and Shoulderstand are not recommended. However, Handstands, Right-Angle Handstands, Dog Poses, and poses that build upper-body strength without bearing weight on the vulnerable neck vertebrae can be safely learned under the guidance of an instructor.

Preventing Fractures and Falls

It is well-known that older people who have osteoporosis tend to fall more often than their strong-boned counterparts. Failing hearing and eyesight, poor posture with a forward head position, weak muscles, and a lack of balance all converge to increase the likelihood of falling down. A fall that causes a bump on the bottom for a younger person can result in a broken bone for an older person with brittle bones.

According to Mary Schatz, M.D., in a March/April 1988 *Yoga Journal* article on teaching people at risk for osteoporotic fractures, lack of exercise affects coordination as much as it does muscle strength and flexibility. Older, stiffer, less active people tend to not catch themselves as easily when they start to fall. According to Dr. Schatz, "neuro-muscular coordination is also affected by posture. Information about the position of the head is sent to the brain from the joints between the cervical vertebrae. In older people with forward head carriage, this feedback system becomes faulty." In other words, when they stumble, this faulty feedback system prevents them from being able to recover their balance. Every slip becomes a potential disaster.

In addition, yoga improves balance and helps prevent falls and fractures, common among elderly people, by improving coordination, posture, and body mechanics during daily life activities.

Yoga also lessens the degree of trauma if a fall is experienced, because muscle strength and flexibility have been increased. As our muscles grow stronger, they are better able to control and absorb the impact of a fall.

Back Pain, Kyphosis, and Spinal Fractures

Pain in the spine can sometimes be the result of muscle spasms associated with microscopic fractures of the collapsing vertebrae. Pain can be sudden and severe, or chronic and constant. With repeated tiny fractures the vertebrae form wedges—narrow in front, wider in back—resulting in upper-back roundness. This increase in the thoracic curve is known as kyphosis or dowager's hump and includes loss of height.

Yoga's ability to help stooped seniors stand taller was demonstrated in a recent study of older women with kyphosis. Research by Gail Greendale, M.D., a gerontologist at the University of California, Los Angeles (UCLA), found that one-hour yoga sessions twice a week for twelve weeks helped participants increase their height, reduce the forward curvature of their spines, and improve their scores on physical tests that assessed such everyday tasks as walking, rising from a chair, and reaching for an object in front of them. Participants also said the yoga helped reduce pain, improve breathing, and increase endurance. According to Dr. Greendale, "More than 60 percent reported increased feelings of well-being."

Although kyphosis is listed as a significant risk factor for osteoporosis, having kyphosis does not mean you have osteoporosis. Only half of the women suffering from this condition experience fractures, and in those who do, the fractures generally occur first, causing the back to round. According to Dr. Greendale, 30 percent of vertebral fractures are symptomatic (painful). As a woman bends forward to escape the pain, she puts more pressure on the anterior (front) part of her spine and suffers more fractures, creating a domino effect.

In others with kyphosis, the condition may result from poor alignment. Bad posture, a weak shoulder girdle, forward head position, flexed hips, and bent knees all contribute to kyphotic posture. If kyphosis is seen as part posture and part structural curvature in the bone itself, those who have it can at least improve the posture element through yoga.

Yoga Postures Increase Bone Density in the Spine

A study by California State University, Los Angeles, of women ages twenty to seventy has shown that yoga postures significantly increased bone density in the spine. Study sponsor Steven Hawkins, assistant professor of kinesiology and nutritional science, states that doctors had previously thought that only high-impact or heavy-lifting exercises could build bone mass. "For many older people, particularly those who are sedentary, such activities are contraindicated. But yoga is a very gentle form of weight-bearing exercise."

Other pilot studies suggest that yoga improves the actual congruence of joints, undoing the "wear and tear" that causes osteoarthritis. Preliminary studies suggest that the variety of unaccustomed tugs of the sinews and ligaments that take place when practicing yoga can not only arrest, but can reverse osteoporosis.

Yoga Helps Prevent Falls and Fractures

Falls are one of the leading problems facing the older person. Injury from falls can lead to permanent disability, limiting a person's active, independent life. It is estimated that one-third of all persons sixty years old and older suffer falls each year. Indirectly, the fear of falling also lowers a person's quality of life. It's estimated that 20 percent of the elderly who fear falling limit their activities of daily living.

The older population's risk of falling is related to three influences on the aging process: pathology that increases with age, side effects from various medications, and environmental conditions. As people age, changes in vision, gait, posture, hearing, and cognition may increase the incidence of falls. For example, a person may not have the muscle strength or reflex reaction to avoid a fall after impaired vision or an unexpected stumble interferes with his or her ability to avoid an obstacle. The elderly also have a higher incidence of chronic illness—cardiovascular conditions, neurological impairments, psychological disorders, metabolic disorders—that may directly influence a person's functional capabilities. Environmental factors include the person's physical surroundings and medications that put them at risk for falling.

In addition to participating in yoga classes and other activities that improve coordination and balance, making simple changes to one's lifestyle and environment can provide peace of mind and prevent the likelihood of falling.

Researchers at Oregon Health & Science University found that older adults who participated in a weekly yoga class and home practice for six months showed significant improvement in measures of flexibility, balance, and fatigue compared to a control group who didn't practice yoga.

According to neurologist Barry Oken, M.D., who has practiced yoga for fifteen years, "We also demonstrated improvements in forward bending and one-legged standing ability. Such improvements are especially valuable for seniors, since fractures resulting from falls are a leading cause of disability among older adults."

Julie Lawrence, an Iyengar-certified instructor who collaborated with colleague Jane Carlsen to create the yoga class used in the Oregon study, states, "Better posture is another plus. Slumping constricts the internal organs and interferes with respiration, circulation, and digestion. Good alignment helps people breathe better, which has a calming effect on the entire body. Also, just as slumping can reflect and magnify a downbeat emotional state, so good alignment can help you feel more cheerful and energetic."

Helping My Mother After She Fell and Broke Her Thigh Bone

Late one evening, while I was writing this book, my father called to tell me that my mother was in the hospital. I cannot recall ever hearing his voice sound so broken and sad. At first I could not grasp what he was saying—something about "if only I had fixed the hallway carpet."

He was trying to tell me that my eighty-five-year-old mother had slipped and fallen in the hallway just before going to bed. Despite terrible pain she did not grasp the severity of her predicament. She stayed on the floor where she fell and asked my father to prop her leg up with a pillow—not yet realizing that her thigh bone was fractured like an egg shell in twenty places! She waited and hoped the pain would subside. Two hours later, my father finally called the ambulance.

Fortunately I live nearby and the hospital was just minutes away. It gave me a shock to see my mother in a hospital bed. Without her dentures, in her gown, she looked about a hundred years old. She had a morphine drip in one arm, and a urine bag hung by the bed. A machine was monitoring her vital signs. She had surgery the next day.

Osteoporosis is usually associated with broken bones. But, as I saw while taking care of my mother, the broken bone itself was not the biggest problem. My mother's fractured thigh triggered a whole series of events related to the aging process—a downward spiral that could have resulted in spending the rest of her life in a wheelchair.

Already thin before she broke her leg, she lost her appetite and began to look as if she were wasting away. When you are bedridden, all the systems of the body become weaker and more susceptible to infection and illness. With less exercise, your arteries become less elastic and more prone to injury. Consequently, your immune system is compromised, and you are even more vulnerable to infections and disease.

After surgery to repair the fracture, the bone healed in about six months. I visited her daily throughout this period, at first helping her from the bed to the bedside commode and back. After the doctor and physical therapist instructed her to begin bearing weight on the bone, I encouraged her to stand upright and put weight on the leg, even if only for ten seconds.

At first my mother was understandably afraid to "test" whether her leg could bear weight again. Without the doctor, physical therapist, and our whole family encouraging her, she might never have regained her ability to walk. I made a game out of it and counted to ten . . . next day fifteen . . . then twenty . . . thirty . . . until she could stand for a minute.

Standing itself was the first milestone, then taking two steps from the bed to the bedside commode. Progress was in small increments—two steps, five, ten. It was a happy day when she made it all the way to the backyard with a walker. Gradually she began to get around without a walker, except for long distances on uneven terrain.

By the time she fully recovered, my mother's experience had given me new appreciation for the body's healing power.

ALEXANDRA (SANDRA) PLEASANTS

"It's Hard to Believe I'm Seventy!"

*S*andra Pleasants *is a senior Iyengar yoga teacher who resides and teaches in Virginia.*

It is hard for me to believe that I'm seventy—which seemed so old even when I was fifty. Seventy was something that only happened to my parents. I believe it now only when I look in the mirror. Yet I know women in their eighties who are vibrant and joyous. In that light it seems rather okay to be seventy. I owe my vigor to twenty years of practice of Iyengar yoga.

I recall that Mr. Iyengar said that the right method of doing asana brings lightness and an exhilarating feeling in the body as well as in the mind. Through this method I have found a way to spiritual growth, maturity, and wisdom that I would not have found otherwise. I am fortunate to have been guided and inspired by superior teachers including Geeta, Prashant, and B. K. S. Iyengar, who have dedicated themselves to this demanding yet fulfilling path.

As I was introduced to yoga when I was nearly fifty, I always felt I was playing catch-up. This required daily practice to learn *Adho Mukha Vrksasana* (Handstands) and *Pincha Mayurasana* (Peacock Pose). These two strengthening inverted poses became the root of my practice and my "drug of choice" if I was feeling lonely or depressed. They stood me in good stead for learning more complicated poses.

I set myself the goal of learning by the age of sixty to drop back into a backbend unaided. I missed the goal by several months, but I had established a routine of practicing backbends with some advanced students for about three hours every week. We had a wonderful time as we were all learning together. Most of the others were approaching forty, but being twenty years older didn't make a difference.

My practice goals have changed over time in part because of past injuries—but also due to greater maturity and wisdom. Now my aim is to be more present in the simpler asanas and enjoy the "juice" of penetrating each pose. I have been sharing this with my students so that they too can penetrate more deeply.

I have been privileged to be asked by the Department of Physical Medicine and Rehabilitation at the University of Virginia to design and teach several studies. The first was to see if ten weeks of yoga could influence the gait of people over sixty. This was a difficult assignment. Yoga works on the whole body and mind, and to limit it to something narrowly measurable was challenging. The participants had to practice twenty minutes a day and come to class twice a week. It was exciting to see the changes that took place from such a concentrated effort.

The next study was for people with Parkinson's disease. I had not worked with this population before, and it was wonderful to see how simple poses and some mindfulness could impact these people so profoundly. Many of the students had severe limitations, but their joy in their progress was infectious. At the end of the series of lessons, two of the students serenaded us on fiddle and banjo. *(See Sandra's observations on teaching people with Parkinson's at the end of Chapter 9.)*

My greatest joy at present is in teaching teachers. In this way I know that the Iyengar tradition will reach far beyond my sphere of influence and will empower many others to place yoga at the forefront of their lives.

CHAPTER 6

Yoga Relief for Arthritis

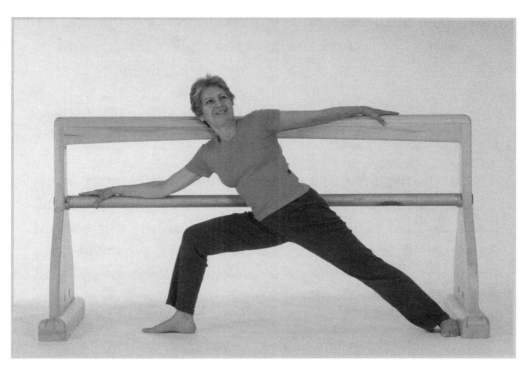

Extended Side-Angle Pose with the horse helps remove stiffness from the joints.

The mind plays a very important role in your perception of pain and also the progression of your arthritis. And when patients are more stressed, when they're depressed, when their muscles are tight, they tend to have more pain. A lot of patients increase pain medication because of stress. Yoga tends to decrease stress and depression, and it lengthens the muscles to help ease pain. And yoga's positive impact on the nonphysical aspects of a person can also produce a very real physical benefit for someone coping with arthritis.

James McKoy, M.D., rheumatologist, quoted in
Shelly Morrow, "Joint Benefits," *Yoga Journal*

At the time that I became interested in yoga, I was helping a woman in her seventies who was immobilized in her wheelchair by arthritis. Long before I understood the degree to which yoga can rehabilitate the body, I was helping people who were unable to dress, bathe, or feed themselves independently due to the pain and stiffness in their joints. This has helped me understand the extreme suffering that can be inflicted by arthritis.

Back then, people with joint pain and swelling were advised by doctors not to move! The thinking was, "If it hurts, don't move it." We now know that arthritis can be influenced in a positive way by movement.

When someone comes to me with arthritis, I encourage them to learn how to practice yoga safely with the support of props.

I have seen what can happen if they do not take their joints through the full range of movement. Where arthritis is concerned, I pull out all the stops in using props! The yoga horse, wall ropes, bolsters, straps, and blankets give the person new hope and confidence and replace fear with a sense of freedom.

An Overview of Arthritis

Inflammation is a natural response to tissue irritation or damage; it causes swelling, redness, heat, and loss of function. The word *arthritis* means "inflammation of the joints," and the pain, swelling, and stiffness that result can lead to immobilization. In extreme cases, people with arthritis are no longer able to live independently.

This chronic health condition is the leading cause of disability in the United States, second only to heart disease as a cause of work disability. It is so common in our culture that most people consider the pain and discomfort it brings to be a normal part of aging. In the United States alone, over 43 million men and women suffer from joint pain caused by arthritis. Eighty-five percent of people sixty-five years and older show evidence of arthritis on x-rays and experience symptoms of pain and stiffness. Arthritis makes normal activities increasingly painful and difficult and diminishes or destroys the quality of life.

Modern medicine recognizes more than a hundred varieties of conditions that produce deterioration in joint structures. The common thread among these conditions is that they all affect the musculoskeletal system. Arthritis-related joint problems may include pain, stiffness, inflammation, and damage to joints. Joint weakness, instability, and visible deformities may occur, depending on the location of the joint involved.

Arthritis is classified into two main types. *Rheumatoid arthritis* is a chronic inflammatory disorder, resulting in stiffness in the joints and muscles, joint erosion, and pain. *Osteoarthritis* is a degenerative disorder that erodes the cartilage in joints, which leads to bones rubbing together. Osteoarthritis frequently occurs in people who are overweight or whose joints are painful from extreme overuse.

In spite of the prevalence of arthritis, be careful not to jump to the conclusion that your achy joints are necessarily due to this condition. Overuse and injuries can also result in tendonitis, bursitis, carpal tunnel syndrome, and other fairly common conditions that are unrelated to arthritis.

Arthritis and Exercise

Most of us respond to pain that occurs during movement by keeping still. However, we now know that inactivity is one of the worst responses for someone with arthritis. To remain healthy, muscles and joints must move and bear weight or they will lose strength. This weakness, coupled with joint swelling, will make the joints unstable. Joints in this condition are vulnerable to dislocation, increased injury and pain. Thus, regular gentle movement helps to reduce pain and to maintain mobility.

Physical movement promotes health in many systems of the body. It increases circulation, which in turn reduces swelling and promotes delivery of oxygen and nutrients to the tissues.

With immobilization, a cycle of deterioration begins.

Because movement is crucial to so many physiological processes, the arthritic person's overall health tends to deteriorate without it. The normal functioning of the immune system declines, infections and illnesses occur, and the person often becomes frustrated and depressed. This cycle is self-perpetuating.

Physicians are increasingly advising regular gentle exercise for people with arthritis because it tones muscles and reduces stiffness in joints. Yoga is an ideal form of exercise for this because its movements are fluid and adaptable. Yoga loosens muscles that have been tightened by inactivity, stress and tension. In yoga we progress gradually, beginning with simple stretches and strengthening poses and advancing to more difficult postures only as we become stronger and more flexible.

If necessary, you can begin with gentle movements while sitting in a chair or lying on the floor. You can gradually add weight-bearing standing postures, with the help of a wall or table, wall ropes, chairs, blocks, and other props.

Practicing yoga can help improve respiration throughout the day. Calm, slow, rhythmic breathing helps to release both physical and emotional tension by flooding the body and brain with oxygen. The regular, daily practice of deep relaxation is restorative to every cell of the body.

I encourage those of you with arthritis to seek the help of an experienced teacher who can help you learn to distinguish between good pain and bad pain and to make yoga part of your daily routine.

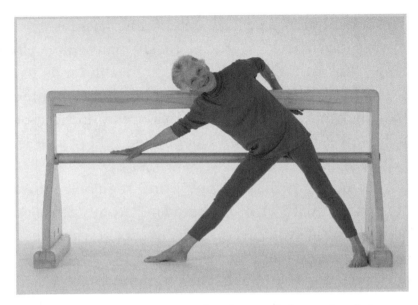

Triangle Pose with the horse, upper hand around the top bar helps open the shoulder joint. The hand on the lower bar lengthens the torso.

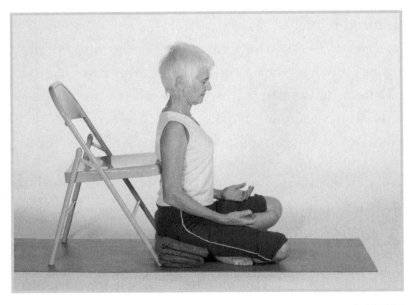

Seated Cross-Legged Pose, Easy Pose, **Sukhasana.** *Sitting on a folded blanket against the edge of a chair helps keep your back straight and hips mobile.*

Yoga and Pain

According to director Lonnie Zeltzer, M.D., who is also a professor of pediatrics, anesthesiology, psychiatry, and biobehavioral sciences at the UCLA School of Medicine, "For people with chronic pain, Iyengar is particularly good, because B. K. S. Iyengar has researched and understood the therapeutic benefits of the poses." Iyengar Yoga's use of bolsters, blocks, straps, blankets, and other supportive props also lets them modify the postures for optimal effectiveness. "Using props allows students to work with their pain instead of avoiding it," Zeltzer says. Props also allow people to do poses that would otherwise aggravate rather than help their condition.

Chronic pain—from arthritis, back problems, repetitive stress injuries, and other ailments—is the most common reason people seek medical attention. Specialists in both Eastern and Western medicine, working together, are offering new treatments. Yoga is a crucial part of these new approaches.

Yoga for Arthritis: Psychological Effects

The positive effects yoga can have on mood and overall outlook are especially important to someone with arthritis. Pain and disability can lead to increasing isolation and depression. A yoga class offers positive support and the opportunity to connect with people who are health minded and have experienced the benefits of yoga. Numerous studies emphasize the value of group support in coping with health challenges.

.Walking is the ideal companion to an intelligent, therapeutic stretch-and-strengthen program. The tranquilizing effect of its moderate, rhythmic exercise decreases pain. The movement and weight-bearing aspects of walking improve joint health.

Equally important, walking can take you outdoors, in touch with nature, the greatest of all healers—uplifting to the mind and spirit. Pace yourself, walk where there are places to rest, and stop there when you feel fatigued. Be in the moment and walk with awareness of the beauty around you.

The psychological benefits of experiencing your strength increasing and your stamina improving are also meaningful. The ability to "stand on your own two feet" cannot be overestimated.

Yoga for Arthritis: Guidelines and Cautions

With arthritis, as with any injury or disease, listen to your body with focused attention to avoid injury and determine which movements are most healing. Look for a teacher who is knowledgeable about arthritis and is willing to communicate with your doctor. If you are new to yoga, I recommend a few private lessons if possible so that you can practice at your own pace.

Combining medical evaluation, nutrition, yoga, massage, and other holistic therapies can break the debilitating cycle of arthritis. Yoga helps people with arthritis learn about their physical limitations without being paralyzed by them.

Keep the following guidelines in mind during your yoga practice and during other exercise.

1. **Breathe properly.** Without fully expanding your lungs, the

muscles you are exercising cannot be adequately supplied with oxygen. Holding your breath while stretching inhibits relaxation. Smooth, peaceful, rhythmic breathing through the nose reduces pain and tension and increases the feeling of deep relaxation that follows a yoga session.

2. **Respect pain.** All yoga students, but especially those with arthritis, must learn the difference between the beneficial feeling of muscles stretching and the pain that signals harm. They must distinguish between the normal discomfort of moving stiff joints and the pain caused by a destructive movement or an excessive demand on a joint. Sudden or severe pain is a warning. Continuing an activity after such a warning may cause joint damage.

    In general, if pain lasts more than two hours after an activity, ask a teacher who understands good alignment to check how you are practicing. Try moving more slowly and practicing more regularly under the guidance of a knowledgeable teacher.

3. **Balance work and rest.** Balancing activity and rest applies to yoga as well as to daily activities. Do not exercise to the point of fatigue. Stop before you are exhausted! Weakened, fatigued muscles set the stage for joint instability and injury. Balance your active yoga session with yoga's deeply relaxing restorative poses. Restorative poses will help your internal healing processes to work. If you are fatigued, practice restorative poses first. You will benefit more from active poses if you are well rested.

4. **Maintain muscle strength and range of motion.** There is

no set answer to the perennial question "How long should I stay in the pose?" Stay long enough so that a healthy change has been made but not so long that your body stiffens from staying in a position too long.

5. **Practice with awareness.** Avoid mechanical repetitions and counting while exercising. Watch the flow of your breath and your body's response to a particular pose or exercise. Learn to tune into what your body is telling you.

6. **Learn to use yoga props.** Props allow you to hold poses longer so you can experience their healing effects. The use of props helps improve blood circulation and breathing capacity. By supporting the body in a yoga posture, props allow the muscles to lengthen in a passive, nonstrenuous way.

People with arthritis may already be quite stiff by the time they start yoga. Props allow them to practice poses they would ordinarily have difficulty in doing. Props help conserve energy and allow people to practice more strenuous poses without overexerting themselves.

Yoga for Arthritic Hips, Knees, and Hands

The areas most commonly affected by arthritis are the hips, knees, and hands. With decreased movement, the muscles and soft tissues around the hip shorten, putting additional wear and tear on the gliding surfaces. If a person becomes more sedentary in an effort to minimize pain, bones and cartilage receive less weight-bearing stimulation. Bone spurs may even develop to further limit movement.

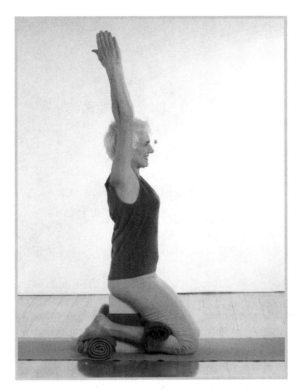

Hero or Heroine Pose, **Virasana.** *In this version of the classic pose, props make the posture easier for those with stiff hips, knees, or ankle joints by using rolled or folded blankets under the ankles and tops of the feet and the backs of the knees and a stack of wood and foam blocks or a bolster under the buttocks.*

Lack of exercise also weakens the thigh and calf muscles. Their strength provides stability and support for the knee. When the soft tissues of the joint swell, this causes compression and reduces space in the joint even further.

Standing poses, such as the Warrior II Pose, are crucial for stretching and building supportive strength in the hips, buttocks, and thighs. Moving the head of the femur in the hip socket helps distribute synovial fluid, thus lubricating the joint and all points of contact.

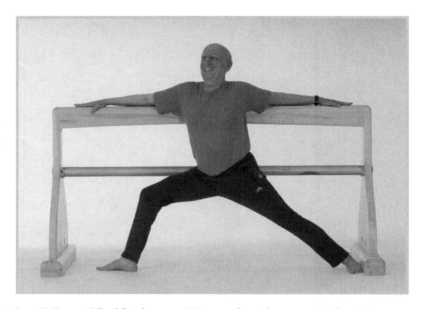

Warrior II Pose, **Virabhadrasana II,** *can first be practiced with support to strengthen leg muscles. Weak muscles are considered a risk factor for osteoarthritis. Weakness is often present before osteoarthritis develops and can contribute to its progression. Be especially aware of weakness in the quadriceps, the large frontal thigh muscles: The weaker the quadriceps, the higher the risk of developing osteoarthritis in the knee.*

The same standing poses recommended for hips are also critical for knee rehabilitation. They create more space in the knee joint for synovial fluid circulation and develop the strength of the thigh and calf muscles for better support.

Yoga Stretching Positions for the Wrists and Hands

Yoga postures such as Downward-Facing Dog Pose require flexibility and strength in the hands and wrists. A careful, gradual approach will allow most students with arthritis to practice such poses in a manner that rehabilitates the joints and does not exacerbate existing problems.

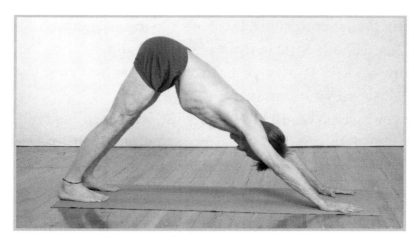

Downward-Facing Dog Pose. Yoga has kept Jim's joints open and functional in spite of osteoarthritis. Practice with the hands on a chair or blocks if your wrists or shoulders are very stiff. Downward-Facing Dog Pose helps relieve arthritis of the shoulders, elbows, wrists, and fingers.

Students with wrist problems can start with positions in which little weight is placed on the hands, such as spending a few minutes simply on hands and knees. If your wrists are already sore or injured, you may need to wait and allow the inflamed tissues to heal. It may take up to several weeks for pain and soreness to subside. Each situation is different.

When I see that a student's hands are already so stiff that they can no longer place their hands flat on a wall or floor, I usually have them try Half Dog Pose with a table or chair and Hanging Downward-Facing Dog Pose with wall ropes. Then they can begin gently stretching the wrists and gradually reintroducing weight bearing in simple positions, such as getting on hands and knees.

When on your hands and knees, you can vary the degree of extension of your wrists. If placing the heels of your hands directly below your shoulders feels too intense, you can move your hands out a little in front of your shoulders to reduce the amount of extension, or you can simply position your knees a little closer to your hands.

As your wrists gradually stretch out, with increased range of motion and endurance, you can put more weight onto them by lifting your knees and straightening your legs into Downward-Facing Dog Pose. People with arthritis may find it especially helpful to begin with modified versions of Upward- and Downward-Facing Dog Pose using a chair (see Chapter 3).

Many of my older students routinely place a folded or a rolled-up sticky mat or a wedge under the heels of the hands to reduce the angle of extension of the wrist in Upward- and Downward-Facing Dog Pose and Plank Pose. A foam-covered yoga prop, or Gripitz (see page 51), also allows the wrists to be in a neutral position.

In addition, working with the alignment of your shoulders, arms, and hands helps take strain off your wrists. Instead of taking all the weight on the heels of the hands, press down with the knuckles where the fingers join the palms. Stretch the fingers forward, and at the same time visualize lifting the fore-arms up and out of the wrists. Apply this action whenever you're bearing weight on the hands.

Caution: *If you have serious wrist problems due to arthritis or previous fracture or surgery sites that are still stiff and painful, please consult your healthcare provider before attempting weight-bearing poses.*

When arthritis develops in the hands, their normal move-ments are altered and the fingers begin to slant outward toward the side of the hand. As swelling overstretches the joint-stabilizing structures, inflammation often causes dislocation. Frequently, the fingers and wrists become discolored and deteriorate. Sometimes muscular shortening makes it impossible to open the hand fully or to separate the fingers. Swelling in the wrist can cause pain and numbness in the hand.

In the following exercises, hands and wrists should not be placed in any position that accentuates or encourages deformity. Every movement should be designed to move the hand back toward normal.

INSTRUCTIONS

Namaste (Prayer) Position

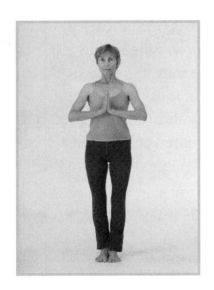

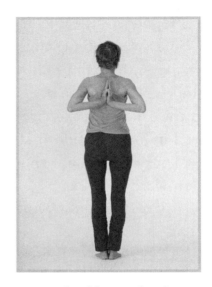

Namaste, *hands in Prayer Position in front of chest.*

As your shoulders and wrists become more flexible, you can gradually learn to practice Prayer Position with the hands in back.

- Sit or stand tall and press your palms together in front of your chest in prayer position. Press the heels of the hands together with your fingers pointing up while gently pressing your hands toward the waist.

- Spread and stretch your fingers as wide apart as possible. To effectively stretch your wrists, do not let the heels of the hands come apart. If you practice this position regularly for a minute or two several times a day, it will stretch the muscles in the hands and help remove stiffness in the fingers. This will help prepare you for weight bearing on the hands and wrists in such poses as Downward-Facing Dog.

• With each repetition, press the heels of the hands, palms, and fingers together more firmly. Encourage the stretched fingers to move more toward the thumb, and the thumbs more toward the chest. Hold this position for several smooth, peaceful, full breaths. Release the pressure, but keep the hands together for a few more breaths. Then repeat the effort three or four times.

• Continue to increase your awareness in this simple but effective stretch. Firmly and evenly press the palms together, especially the parts of the palm at the base of each finger and heel of the hand. Now, instead of keeping the fingers connected, stretch the fingers backward, away from each other, gradually increasing the V-shaped space between them. Again encourage the fingers to move toward the thumb side of the hand, and hold for several breaths. Release and repeat three or four more times.

JIM JACOBS

Yoga Keeps My Body Free in Spite of Arthritis

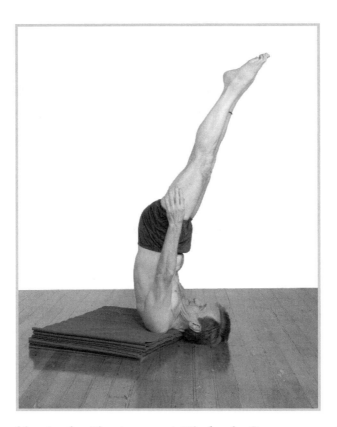

Shoulderstand without support, **Niralamba Sarvangasana II.**

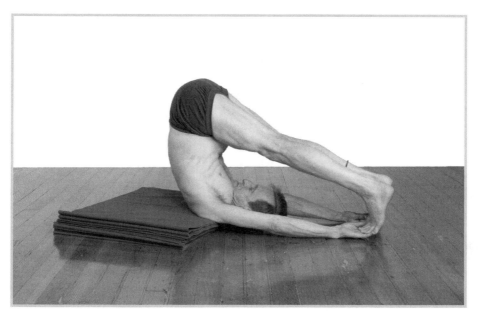

Plow Pose, **Halasana,** *feet on floor, variation with hands holding feet.*

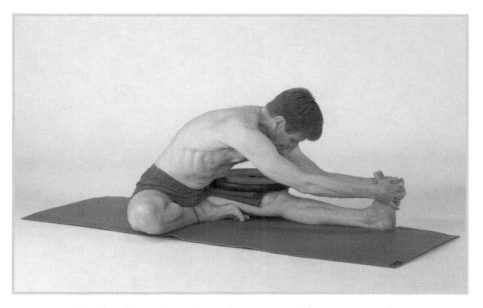

Head to Knee Pose, **Janusirsasana,** *with support on leg.*

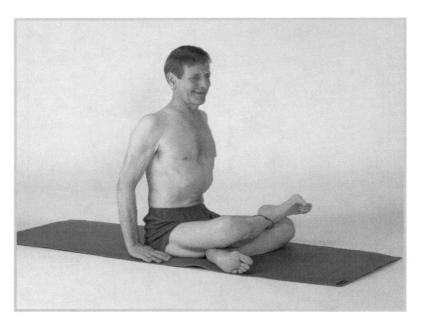

Hip Opener, Lotus Pose preparation.

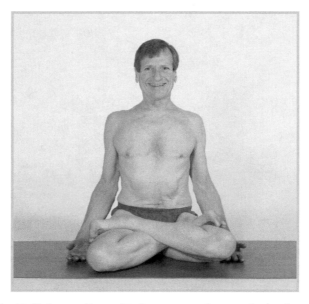

Jim Jacobs in Full Lotus Pose, **Padmasana,** *the symbol of creation and a classic pose for meditation.*

*B*orn *in 1941, Jim Jacobs has practiced Iyengar yoga for over twenty years.*

I've been physically active throughout my adult life. At age thirty I began to experience arthritic symptoms that were diagnosed a number of years later as symptoms of osteoarthritis. Apparently, I am genetically predisposed to early osteoarthritis. I began a serious practice of Iyengar yoga twenty years ago at age forty-five, which greatly lessened my arthritic symptoms and has continued to do so.

At fifty-eight I began experiencing weakness in my left foot and pain in my left buttock and leg. This was the result of severe osteoarthritis, as well as scoliosis in my lumbar spine. After three years of trying conservative treatments, it became clear that the deterioration and stenosis (narrowing) in my lumbar spine were increasing and would lead to increasing dysfunction over time.

At sixty-one I had a very major back reconstruction: fusion of the four deteriorating vertebrae and removal of the bony overgrowths narrowing the spinal canal and pinching the nerves. This required two operations, each over five hours long and done five days apart. I was in the hospital for two weeks and spent the better part of a year fully recovering.

I consider the surgery a total success: My foot strength came back, my leg pain was cured, and I have resumed all of my favorite activities. I even went scuba diving ten months after the surgery. I now have much less lumbar scoliosis and a normal lumbar curve. My spine is rigid from the pelvis to the top of L2. However, I more than compensate for this lack of flexibility in the lower spine by my flexibility in the hip and upper back that I attribute to my yoga practice.

My spinal surgeon believes, as do I, that yoga kept me functional for many years before my surgery. The rheumatologist who diagnosed my osteoarthritis believes that yoga has kept my joints as open and functional as they are.

To me yoga is a daily gift—an experimental approach to being in the body, accepting limitation, and expanding areas of function and freedom.

CHAPTER 7

Get Hip About Your Hips: Yoga and Hip Replacement Surgery

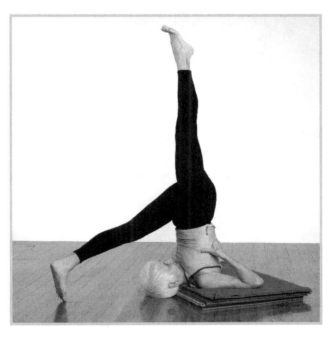

One-Legged Shoulderstand, **Eka Pada Sarvangasana,** *works the hip socket without wearing it out. If your hamstrings are too tight to allow the bottom leg to reach the floor without sagging your spine, place the bottom foot on a chair.*

*I thought hip replacements were for older people
or those who had let themselves go.*

Forty-nine-year-old triathlete,
after hip replacement surgery

T he first time a student in her mid-seventies informed me that she had an artificial hip, I had only a vague idea what that was. Until a few years ago, I thought that joint replacement was something that older people did as a last resort to keep themselves mobile and out of a wheelchair.

I now know that total hip replacement (THR) surgery is considered one of the most important surgical advances of the twentieth century. Also known as *hip arthroplasty*, hip replacement surgery replaces a diseased hip with a cemented or uncemented artificial hip.

Hip replacement surgery is becoming more and more common. Open up the health section of any newspaper or magazine and you will likely see an aging athlete in an advertisement for "Same-Day Hip Replacement." Artificial joints are now made from longer-lasting materials, such as titanium, that look luminous and futuristic in photographs. In fact, one of my students commented, "They look so beautiful it makes you want to run out and get one!"

More than 600,000 hip and knee replacements are performed in the United States every year. As baby boomers age, the number of replacements is expected to increase dramatically.

According to the American Academy of Orthopaedic Surgeons, the biggest growth in joint replacement surgeries is occurring in people between the ages of fifty and fifty-nine. Today, one out of every three knee and hip replacements are performed on people in this age group.

Over the last twenty-five years, major advancements in hip replacement have greatly improved the outcome of this surgery. Total hip replacement relieves pain from most kinds of hip arthritis and thereby improves the quality of life for the large majority of patients who undergo the operation.

Better-quality replacement devices, smaller incisions, advances in anesthesia, improved pain management, and faster recoveries are making joint replacements more tolerable and acceptable. These advances allow many people to go home the same day of surgery or within two or three days, using a walker or crutches.

Physical therapy and yoga both help to optimize the effects of the surgery and to improve outcomes. Stretching, strengthening, and stabilization exercises are critical for improving both short- and long-term functional recovery.

The Price of High-Impact Exercise

Although age, obesity, and arthritis are still the leading reasons why people need new knees and hips, a growing number of younger and fitter people are finding they need new joints as well.

Orthopedic surgeons are seeing an increasing number of younger adults whose extremely active lifestyles put high demands on their joints. These active baby boomers may not have heart disease, stroke, diabetes, or the other diseases associated with an inactive lifestyle, but, in the process of all that running on pavement, their joints take a pounding. While running and other demanding sports don't cause arthritis, they are accelerators.

Though elite athletes may be fast, skilled, and strong enough to juggle Hummers, the price they pay comes later, because their bodies (even if they compete in non-contact sports) can't handle the constant battering. We know it's a hard concept to imagine when today's athletes look as if they're chiseled out of granite. But the reality is that excessive exercise is like a category 5 hurricane to your body. The more pounding you take— even if you aren't a super athlete—the greater the chance that the foundation of your house (your bones and joints) is going to be reduced to rubble.

Mehmet Oz, M.D., and **Michael Roizen, M.D.,**
You: The Owner's Manual

Hello, Hip Replacement

A painful hip can severely affect the ability to do many of the normal activities that most of us take for granted. Typically, the first sign of trouble is when you feel pain in and around a joint. Unlike pain from an injury or soreness from too much weekend exercise, which goes away in a few days, this kind of joint pain persists and keep coming back. Recurring or constant pain is a likely sign that you should consult an orthopedist.

Yoga will not necessarily prevent the need for hip replacement, but a balanced yoga practice can keep a joint healthier for a longer period of time. A yoga practice prior to hip surgery prepares the body for the surgical impact. Yoga after the surgery can help with restoring mobility and coping with pain and emotions that accompany any trauma to the body.

In my classes, no one ever dislocated his or her artificial hip, because we followed some simple guidelines: (1) focusing on regaining normal range of motion (functional movement) and avoiding extreme positions; (2) encouraging students to practice the healing standing poses with the support of the yoga horse, walls, ropes, tables, and chairs; and (3) pacing the class slow enough so that students feel unpressured and unrushed and have time to breathe slowly, practice peacefully, and listen to their bodies' feedback.

Some teachers offer yoga and hip replacement workshops, which are designed to address the questions and concerns of yoga teachers and students: post–hip replacement hazards and limitations, as well as the necessary adaptations of yoga poses for safety and strengthening.

Recovery from hip replacement surgery can be both physically and mentally challenging. A yoga program adapted to the individual offers all the elements needed on the road to recovery after surgery: good posture, balance, stability, strength, and flexibility.

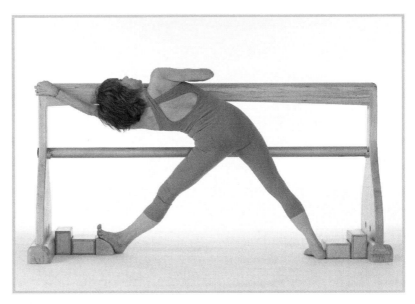

The model, Nora Burnett, has had two recent hip replacements. A block under the front foot helps take the load off the sore joint.

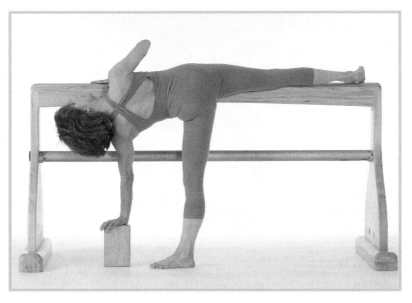

Half-Moon Pose with the support of the horse.

Heal Your Hips

Ask your doctor lots of questions. Be skeptical. Take advantage of the Internet to learn as much as you can about your hip condition. Ask your surgeon to go over your X-rays with you. Don't let him just read you the report. You need to learn to read them and watch the progression of your hip condition yourself. Keep your own X-rays so if you change doctors you'll have all your X-rays together in one place showing the progression over time.

Robert Klapper, M.D., author of Heal Your Hips,
Co-Director of The Joint Replacement Institute and Clinical Chief
of Orthopedics, Cedars-Sinai Medical Center in Los Angeles

Reasons for Hip Replacement and Alternatives

The most common reason for hip replacement surgery is the wearing down of the hip joint caused by osteoarthritis. Other conditions, such as rheumatoid arthritis, injury, and bone tumors, may also lead to the breakdown of the hip joint and the need for hip replacement surgery.

According to the Centers for Disease Control, approximately 65 million Americans suffer from some form of arthritis or chronic joint symptom. The hip is the second most commonly affected large joint, after the knee. More than a hundred different conditions cause joint inflammation and can lead to permanent destruction of the weight-bearing surface of the hip.

Alternatives to hip replacement surgery are available. Medical doctors might suggest a walking aid, such as a cane.

They might also recommend medications to treat inflammation in the hip joint and to help relieve pain. Physical therapy and a yoga-based exercise program can help to strengthen muscles around the hip joint and relieve pain.

Surgical Nuts and Bolts

The hip is basically a ball-and-socket joint. It links the ball at the head of the thigh bone (the femur) with the cup-shaped socket (the acetabulum) in the pelvis.

In traditional hip replacements, doctors replace the top of the femur with a metal ball and remove portions of the damaged hip socket. Resurfacing, a less invasive procedure, is available today and involves coating the ball of the femur with metal instead of completely removing it. Resurfacing is meant for people with limited bone damage, as determined by an orthopedic surgeon.

Recovery from Hip Replacement Surgery

Physical therapy typically starts the day after surgery. A physical therapist will teach you exercises, such as contracting and relaxing certain muscles that can strengthen the muscles, bones, and joint around the artificial hip. Because the new hip has a limited range of movement, the physical therapist also will teach you proper techniques for simple activities of daily living, such as bending and sitting, to prevent injury to the new hip.

Most patients will walk with a walker or crutches for four to six weeks. Many will use a cane for another four to six weeks after that. Regaining normal function takes about three to six months. As in bone fractures, healing time for older persons will typically take longer than for younger persons.

Appropriate physical activity can reduce joint pain and stiff-ness and increase flexibility and muscle strength. Unless the hip joints are exercised in all directions, problems will emerge, including stiffness, pain, and muscle shortening. It is also important during recovery to meet the challenge of regaining proprioception: the body's ability to recognize and correct posture and balance.

People with a hip replacement should avoid certain high-impact activities for the rest of their lives. Running, basket-ball, tennis, and other high-impact activities should be avoided to minimize loosening and wearing of the joint. Activities and yoga postures that cause internal rotation or excessive external rotation of the affected joint increase the likelihood of hip dislocation.

Yoga for Recovery from Hip Replacement Surgery

A modified yoga practice, combined with physical therapy and medical care, can greatly facilitate the recovery process. Progressively integrating yoga into the recovery plan is excel-lent for regaining both stability and functional (normal) range of motion, maintaining the health of connective tissue, addressing the emotional aspects of recovery, and supporting the body holistically.

Most basic postures can be modified or adapted to safely support hip replacement recovery. As strength and range of motion improve, additional poses can be added.

A timeline for beginning a practice is very individual, depending on the person's recovery progress and condition prior to surgery. Extreme actions can cause dislocation and can make the shaft or head of the artificial femur impinge on the rim of the hip socket, thus damaging the joint.

Individuals with yoga experience and those who use yoga's therapeutic techniques experience immediate gains in strengthening and healing. A consistent practice and working with a well-trained teacher or therapist who can monitor alignment and provide feedback are most supportive.

Note: *Yoga supports the body's innate healing intelligence. As you read the following guidelines, keep in mind that each individual's circumstances are unique, and the time it takes to recover varies from person to person.*

Yoga for New Hips: Guidelines and Cautions

1. **Give yourself time to rest, recover, and heal.** Practice Deep Relaxation Pose and appropriate restorative poses daily. Practice poses that relieve neck and shoulder tightness. Think of your practice as post-surgery stress relief.

2. **Remember that your whole body is connected!** This is a good time for a massage. Receiving bodywork on the neck, soles of the feet, and other areas will help the rest of your body to relax and heal.

3. **Take extra care in aligning the feet and legs in all postures.**

4. **Be alert not to overdo it when exercising uninjured areas.** Use the wall, wall ropes, and chair or another sturdy support like the yoga bar (tressler) to stabilize and protect the

hip joint, and to move in and out of standing poses safely.

5. **Actively exercise the muscles and tendons to strengthen them, prevent further damage and allow healing for the tissues around the prosthesis.**

6. **Partial hip replacements are much less prone to dislocation than total replacements.** The same general precautions apply, but you should be able to safely do more movements.

7. **Ask your doctor which actions are beneficial and which ones you should avoid.** His or her recommendations may differ from the general advice in this chapter.

Your yoga practice will help you to regain and maintain a normal, healthy range of motion. A consistent home practice, paired with classes, will contribute to the stabilization of the hips, bringing balance and assisting successful healing of muscles, ligaments, tendons, and other connective tissues around the prosthesis.

Yoga Poses for Hip Students

A modified yoga practice prior to surgery helps prepare the body for the impact of the surgery. After the surgery, yoga helps with stamina, restoration, and pain management, and even addresses the emotional component that accompanies any trauma to the body.

To understand contraindicated movements for hip replacement, learn as much about your surgery as possible. Two approaches to hip replacement surgery are possible: anterior (from the front) and posterior (from the rear). This distinction, which describes whether the surgical entry (incision) is made from the front or the back of the body, has important implications for recovery, future movement, and your yoga practice.

Avoid extreme hip actions in any direction. Practice yoga with the "goal" of establishing functional range of motion.

Practice standing poses with caution and adequate support, and be conservative about how far you step your feet apart. Use the horse, walls, chairs, counters, or other stable supports for standing poses for additional stability and security when you practice. Experiment with a less wide stance, placing the feet closer together than usual, and bend the knee less, being careful that the knee does not go past the heel and that you keep your thigh (femur) straight. All the principles of good alignment are extra important after hip replacement.

To reduce the risk of dislocation, it is crucial to stabilize the hip joint by strengthening the muscles that cross it. Almost all standing postures are good for this, practiced as described to avoid extreme actions and overstretch and to limit specific movements that make dislocation more likely.

Postures that strengthen muscles in the backs of the thighs (hamstrings), in the fronts of the thighs (quadriceps), in the buttocks (gluteals), and around the hips may be especially helpful after posterior surgery. Backbends such as Bridge Pose, *Setu Bandha Sarvangasana*, strengthen the hamstrings, quadriceps, and gluteals. Tree Pose, *Vrksasana*, and other one-leg standing poses strengthen the hip. You can also practice Standing Big Toe Pose with the lifted leg supported on a table, counter, or yoga horse.

Sitting upright in simple seated poses with the legs straight, such as Seated Wide-Angle Pose, *Upavistha Konasana,* are generally beneficial. Poses such as Seated or Lying-Down Bound-Angle Pose are also generally beneficial and can easily be modified by bringing the feet less close to the body and supporting the legs with folded blankets.

Lying-down poses are generally safe, as long as extreme movements are avoided. Inverted poses, such as Legs Up the Wall Pose, will help to relax and revitalize the whole body.

Private yoga lessons can be very helpful during the recovery process. Experienced teachers working with students they knew prior to surgery can usually accommodate individual needs in a group setting, but at least one private session before joining a group after surgery makes good sense. If you are the owner of a new hip (or pair of hips) make sure you fully understand both the recommended and contraindicated movements for your surgery, especially in the first year or two of recovery.

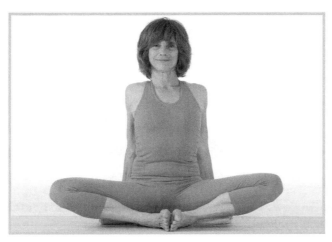

Bound-Angle Pose may feel more comfortable with the feet further away from the body. Our hip joints become stiff through incorrect use, or under or over use. Ease of movement of the hip joints is especially important in later life when movement tends to become slow and difficult.

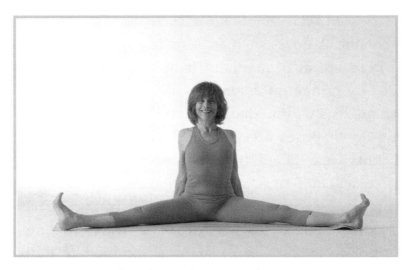

Seated Wide-Angle Pose. Before surgery,
Nora could barely take her feet wide apart.

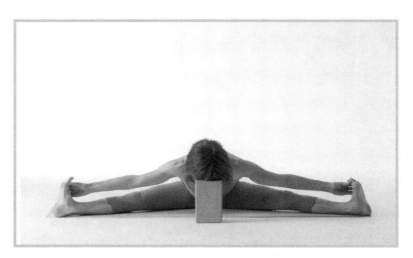

Seated Wide-Angle Pose, bending forward from hip hinge. Follow bent-knee
poses with poses where the legs are straight.

NORA BURNETT
I Danced All Through My Youth

*N*ora Burnett is a fifty-seven-year-old yoga teacher. At the time the photos of Nora were taken, she was a year and three months past the first (left hip) surgery and eight months past the second surgery.

I danced all through my youth, performing and teaching in my twenties and thirties. I also taught high impact aerobics. There is a significant history of arthritis in my family.

I had lived for a long time with aching hips, which very gradually progressed to extremely limited range of motion, a very compromised gait, serious postural distortion, and persistent pain.

It took me a long time to come to terms with having surgery, especially since I'm relatively young to have hip replacements. I am still integrating and re-educating my body post-surgery.

I work a lot on simple poses to regain overall strength, which diminished while I was in pain; more symmetry through the spine and pelvis; and, of course, stability and flexibility in the hips. The trestler (horse) has been invaluable, especially in lifting the load off the hips with my arms while the tissues have been healing and the new joints gaining stability.

I have been very gradually using less support. I had to learn to back off from doing more, and not irritate the joints prior to surgery, and to re-strengthen without pushing too far. My hips are great teachers, the lessons reaching far beyond the obvious physical concerns.

I'm still integrating these new metal hips into how I function, and I'm grateful to be able to walk well, not be in pain, and continue to practice and teach yoga.

A Yoga Teacher's Hip Replacement

*O*ne of my yoga teacher friends shared her hip replacement story with me a week after she had surgery.

I only had one hip replaced: the left side. It has been quite a journey for me since I was in excruciating pain—*constantly*—for four months before the surgery. This whole ordeal has changed me forever in so many ways, and I do have a lot of thoughts about it all.

I was diagnosed with degenerative osteoarthritis. I was in shock and it totally freaked me out. I think I was also in denial. From the x-rays it was easy to see that I had absolutely no cartilage in my left hip and only about half of what I am supposed to have in my right, which I might also have to have replaced in the future.

I am the only active, athletic person in my family. As far as I know there have been no bone problems in any other family members, until me.

Nobody knows exactly what happened to me, including myself, but I have my own theories. I have never ever been a moderate person. When I go for something, I go all the way. For thirty years I practiced yoga on my own for up to four hours a day and taught many classes a week. I also taught aerobics in the seventies, and over the years I have done a lot of dancing. On top of all this, I am an avid hiker.

I am a thin, small-boned woman. So, when I am totally honest with myself, I think I just wore myself out. I think this is a huge lesson in balance for me, which is the *true* yoga. Up until my surgery I kept saying that all I cared about is being able to walk pain free and to take hikes again. I feel certain I will be able to do this.

As for yoga . . . if I can do some basic stretches and simple poses, I will be very happy. I would *love* to be able to develop a yoga system for people who have had hip replacement.

Starting Yoga After
Bilateral Hip Replacement

*T*he author of this story wishes to remain anonymous.

I am a cardiology nurse practitioner in my fifties. I was a very flexible, semi-fit individual who enjoyed outdoor exercises, especially walking and biking, until two years prior to my bilateral hip replacement. During those two years my flexibility disappeared and every motion was painful. I counteracted the pain with anti-inflammatory medication, massage, and rest. Even with these measures, I was still struggling on a daily basis with this monster called chronic pain.

After surgery to replace both hips, my pain was almost nil, and I resumed walking and biking. Nevertheless my range of motion and flexibility improved only slightly. I did not take any yoga classes for about two years after surgery. This was due to my uncertainty about how to improve my range of motion, fear of a dislocation, and my limited knowledge about yoga in general. As a result of discussions with expert teachers such as Carol Krucoff, I decided to try gentle yoga. Within three or four weeks my flexibility and range of motion had increased by sixty or seventy degrees!

My wonderful, joyful teacher asks every new student if they have had any previous experience with yoga and if they have any health concerns. When I mentioned I had bilateral hip replacements, she was very supportive and has suggested alternate positions if any of the poses feel uncomfortable.

I am able to practice most of the gentle, level I yoga poses. For sitting poses I either support my knees or just keep my legs straight in front of me. These are some of the "pearls" I have learned in a short time of practice:

- For me the most important lesson is to listen to my body. If a position or stretch feels uncomfortable I reduce it or try another pose. I allow myself to be a beginner and don't push to an extreme of perfection.

- If I can stretch a little farther in the next practice, I try to enjoy how that feels and to notice and be thankful that my flexibility is better. I allow myself to enjoy the small accomplishment of holding a pose a little longer and to marvel with respect at those who are truly the masters.

- I may never be at the level of some of the students with whom I have the honor to share a class. However, we all acknowledge with gratitude that this is a journey and a nonjudgmental process. There is a mutual acceptance within the group that no matter what pose we are in we are all, in one sense, at the same level. For me that is the true essence of yoga.

CHAPTER 8

The Yoga Prescription for a Healthy Heart

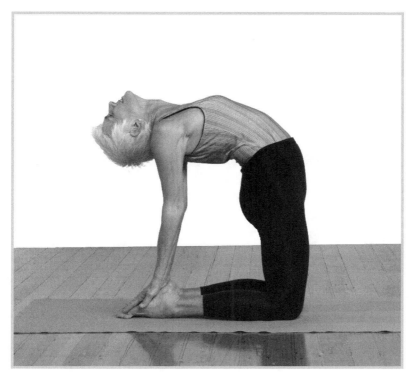

Camel Pose, **Ustrasana,** *increases lung capacity and improves blood circulation to all the organs of the body. If you are recovering from a heart attack, practice this pose with the body supported with props, under the guidance of an experienced instructor.*

We don't know where the soul is in the body . . .
there's actually a piece of tissue in the heart that touches
all four chambers. And the heart really is that entity
for me—it's power, strength, energy and spirit.

Mehmet Oz, M.D., heart surgeon,
Columbia Presbyterian Medical Center,
New York, from his book *Healing from the Heart*

I always look forward to Dr. Mehmet Oz's appearances on *Oprah*. Dr. Oz, one of the nation's leading heart surgeons, is a pioneer in blending Eastern and Western traditions of medicine. Along with Dr. Dean Ornish and some others in the healthcare profession, Dr. Oz is on a mission to teach the world that we can prevent or even reverse heart disease.

Via the magic of modern photography, Dr. Oz has given viewers of *Oprah* amazing tours inside the human body, including unforgettable live images inside the chambers of the beating human heart. Another of Dr. Oz's memorable teaching techniques is to show actual diseased hearts and other organs so that we can see "up close and personal" exactly how our eating habits affect our health.

Dr. Oz describes cardiovascular disease as "the rusting of our arteries. Literally, the tubes that carry nourishment to our different organs are rotting from the inside. And that's not just about dying from heart attacks and strokes. It's about kidney failure and loss of quality of life."

We are all familiar with expressions like "I love you with all my heart," "My heart hurts," "a pain in the heart," and "I feel you in my heart." When we are sad, hurt, angry, or depressed our body responds by slumping forward, tightening, and closing the chest area where the heart is located.

In a yoga class, you are likely to hear the teacher talk about "opening the heart center." While all yoga poses benefit the health of the heart, yoga backbends dramatically stretch and open the chest and heart center. Yoga philosophy and practitioners of mind–body medicine all recognize that the area in the chest where the heart is located, generally referred to as the "heart center," is the place where body, mind, and spirit converge.

Heart disease is highly individual. Someone with relatively little obstruction in the coronary arteries can be incapacitated by chest pains, while another person with more severely obstructed arteries may not even be aware of a problem. Some people have run marathons with 85 percent of their coronary arteries blocked; others, with no outward sign of arteriosclerosis, have dropped dead of heart attacks. Physical causes alone explain only a portion of heart disease.

William Harvey, the father of modern heart physiology, understood over 300 years ago that the mind and emotions affect the health of the heart. As he put it, "Every affection of the mind that is attendant with either pain or pleasure, hope or fear, is the cause of an agitation whose influence extends to the heart."

It is now widely recognized that emotional and spiritual factors are involved in creating and maintaining heart health. Unresolved emotional and spiritual issues, such as a broken heart, depression, anger, or lack of fulfillment, can physically affect the health of the heart.

Herbert Benson, M.D., first coined the term *relaxation response* in the 1970s to describe the profound physical and mental responses that occur when we consciously relax (also see Chapter 1). Benson was among the first scientists to document yoga's ability to significantly reduce stress, improve health, and benefit the heart.

The practice of yoga encourages us to *observe* our reactions to daily events. Through the process of self-observation, we become aware of the totality of our responses to emotions, such as fear, anger, and anxiety.

The next time you feel angry, try to feel how your digestive system begins to shut down so that blood and energy can be diverted to the large muscles needed for fighting or running. If you are really angry, the arteries in your arms and legs will begin to constrict, and your blood chemistry will change so that clots form more quickly to conserve your blood should you be wounded.

Under conditions of intense chronic stress, even the muscle fibers inside the heart itself can begin to contract so vigorously that the normal architecture of these fibers is disrupted, damaging the heart muscle. To me this is an amazing metaphor: The inability of the heart to relax causes the heart's muscle fibers to constrict to the point that it damages itself— like clenching your fist so hard and for so long that the bones and knuckles in your hand begin to break.

Dean Ornish, M.D.,
Dr. Dean Ornish's Program for Reversing Heart Disease

*When we have no time for yoga,
that's the time for yoga!*

Aadil B. Palkhivala, Director,
Yoga Centers, Bellevue, Washington

Our Heartbeat Responds to
Our Breathing Pattern

Taking time to relax deeply and to reduce stress is not a luxury but a health-promoting and potentially life-extending technique. The breath is the bridge between the body and mind. Our heartbeat responds to our breathing pattern. It gently accelerates when we inhale and slows when we exhale.

The emphasis in yoga on inhaling slowly, gently, without strain and exhaling completely is relaxing for the heart muscle. Begin now to become aware of your breath, and take time to practice slow, gentle, calm, even breathing. It's the first step to feeling more relaxed.

Posture Also Affects Heart Health

Our everyday posture—the way we sit, stand, and walk— affects our respiration, circulation, and heart health. Chronic slouching decreases circulation to all the vital organs.

One of yoga's most immediate effects is improvement in our posture. The body sighs with relief as the chest opens, and the breath flows freely. Standing poses, backbends, and inverted poses open the chest and expand the breathing process. Upward-Facing and Downward-Facing Dog, both from the floor and with the aid of wall ropes, stretch the muscles of the front of the body, expand the chest, increase breathing capacity, and strengthen the back, chest, and shoulder muscles.

Gentle supported backbends and various restorative postures expand the chest, lungs, and rib cage without effort. These passive poses are useful for everyone but are especially recommended after healing from heart surgery. They should be practiced with the guidance of a qualified instructor.

Krishna Raman, M.D., a leading expert and writer on the integration of yoga with Western medicine states the following in *A Matter of Health: Integration of Yoga and Western Medicine for Prevention and Cure*:

> Backbends are particularly important for preventing and relieving coronary problems. Forward bends with support relieve elevated blood pressure. Inversions are very important

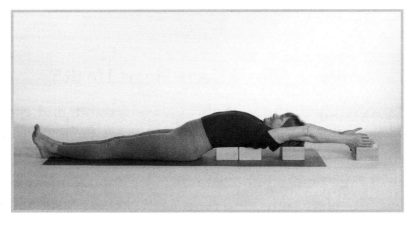

Chest opener, backbend preparation, with blocks.

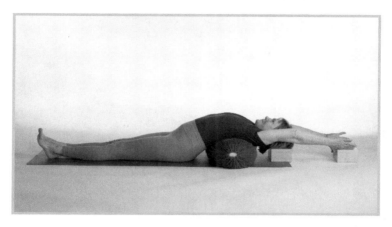

Chest opener, backbend preparation series, with bolster, fingers stretching toward block, variation with block under head.

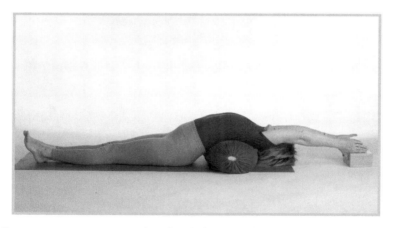

Stretch your arms over your head, while stretching your legs and feet in the opposite direction.

to enhance and maintain a healthy circulatory status. They preserve the integrity of the fascial tissues and relieve stagnation of fluid in the legs. They also prevent generalized water retention, by regularizing the hypothalamus–pituitary axis, which regulates water balance in the body. Inversions give rest to the heart from the strain of gravity.

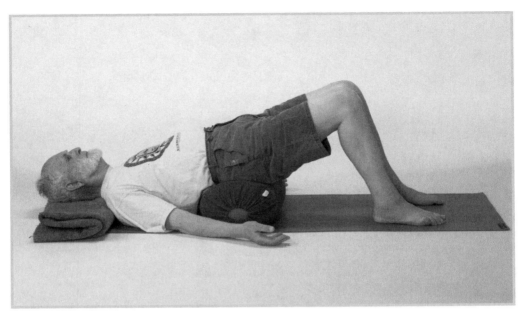

Supported Bridge Pose, folded blanket under head, bolster under lower back.

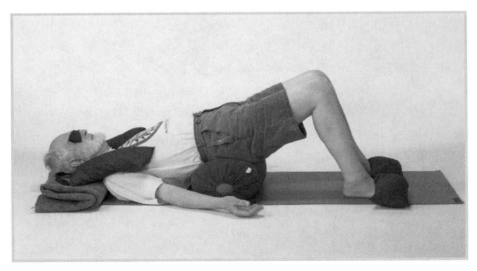

Supported Bridge Pose, sandbags over feet, sandbag over each shoulder and eye bag over eyes, to help the body relax.

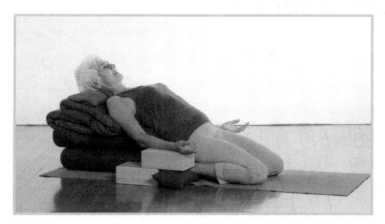

Supported Lying-Down Hero Pose (**Supta Virasana**). *The chest opening in this restful, supported variation of the classic pose is particularly beneficial for the heart. Supported Lying-Down Hero Pose helps prevent arterial blockages by gently massaging and strengthening the heart and increasing coronary blood flow. It stretches the abdomen, aids digestion, and is one of the few poses that can be done after a heavy meal.*

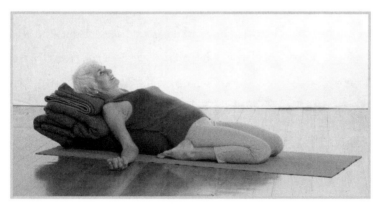

Supported Lying-Down (**Hero**) *Pose,* **Supta Virasana,** *on bolster, head supported palms up.*

Caution: *If you have chest pains (angina) or partially blocked arteries, or are recovering from bypass surgery, practice this pose only under the guidance of a knowledgeable teacher.*

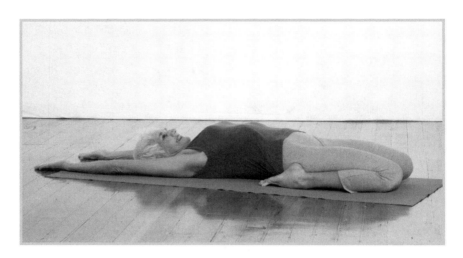

Lying-Down Hero Pose, **Supta Virasana,** *without props, arms stretching back.*

According to Dr. Krishna Raman and other yoga experts, passive, supported backbends, such as *Viparita Dandasana,* gently stretch the heart muscle and the cardiac vessels that supply the heart. This increases blood flow to the heart and helps prevent arterial blockages. Backbends also help maintain the elasticity of blood vessels and force the heart to contract—lengthening cardiac muscle and enhancing blood flow. The most important task of the cardiovascular system is to supply blood to the brain. Inverted poses help strengthen the heart, increase blood flow to the brain, and may prevent the death of brain cells.

Yoga postures also help maintain the elasticity of blood vessels. Passive backbends stretch cardiac vessels. Yoga breathing practices help prevent rhythm disturbances of the heart. Standing poses strengthen cardiac reserves. Forward bends improve the function of the sympathetic nervous system, which in turn affects cardiac nerves. Backbends force the heart to contract, lengthening cardiac muscle, and enhancing blood flow.

Yoga and Hypertension

Nearly 20 percent of adults in the United States have high blood pressure (hypertension). Hypertension is caused by multiple factors, including improper diet, stress, lack of exercise, and excess body fat. It increases the risk of not only hardening of the arteries and heart attacks but also of mini strokes in the brain, which may result in dementia.

A restorative yoga practice is recommended for relieving heart palpitations, breathlessness, regulating blood pressure, and calming the nervous system.

B. K. S. Iyengar on the Heart, Yoga, and Blood Pressure

According to B. K. S. Iyengar, yoga postures can benefit the health of your heart many different ways. Yoga addresses the causes, as well as the effects, of high blood pressure. It calms the mind and regularizes and balances the autonomic nervous system, the center that controls stress. The sympathetic and parasympathetic nervous systems, which are involved in stress reactions, also get stabilized in the practice of asanas, resulting in regulation of blood pressure.

The asanas recommended for regulating blood pressure

include forward bend, supine, sitting, and inverted poses. Forward bend sequences are recommended for people who have high blood pressure. Supported backbends, such as *Viparita Dandasana*, are considered to be the most beneficial asana for low blood pressure.

Forward bends should be practiced with bolsters and blankets. In forward bends, the frontal brain is pacified and blood flow to the brain is regularized. Stress gets released from the eyes, nose, throat, and tongue. Stress, chronic headaches, and eye pain are also reduced.

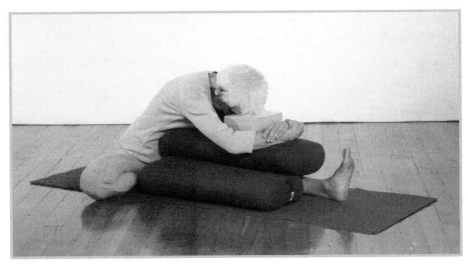

Seated Forward Bend Pose, **Janusirsasana.** *In most mammals, the spine is parallel to the ground and the heart is below the spine. In humans, the spinal column is perpendicular to the ground. Because of our upright position, we are more prone to strain and to diseases of the heart. In Seated Forward Bends, the spine is parallel to the ground so that the heart can rest.*

The sympathetic nervous system gets rested in forward bends, and this has a positive effect on the other body systems. Blood pressure becomes stable when the sense organs, the brain, and the sympathetic nervous system are relaxed. The horizontal position of the spine in these asanas allows the heart to slow down as there is no stress to pump the blood against gravity to the brain. The heart rate slows down, and blood pressure is controlled.

Forward-bending standing poses and Downward-Facing Dog Pose *(Adho Mukha Svanasana)*, have an effect on the nervous system similar to Seated Forward Bends. When these poses are practiced with the head resting on props, the blood flows more freely, and blood pressure becomes stabilized.

People with hypertension often have problems with breathing. Seated poses soften the diaphragm and remove tension from the ribs and the intercostal muscles. This helps the person to breathe easily.

Give Your Heart a Break

The human body is sensitive to the fluctuations of gravity because it consists of about two-thirds water. Sometimes it is helpful to think of your body as a balloon filled with water. To get the water to move around, you could shake up the balloon by running, jogging, or dancing. With yoga's inverted postures, you could turn the balloon upside down. Inverted poses directly benefit the heart by increasing the volume of blood coursing through it.

When the human body inverts, tissue fluids in the lower extremities drain far more effectively than when one is asleep. As David Coulter, Ph.D., writes in *Anatomy of Hatha Yoga*, "If you can remain in an inverted posture for just 3 to 5 minutes, the blood will not only drain quickly to the heart, but tissue fluids will flow more efficiently into the veins and lymph channels of the lower extremities and of the abdominal and pelvic organs, facilitating a healthier exchange of nutrients and wastes between cells and capillaries."

Inverting gives the heart a break. The heart works incessantly to ensure that freshly oxygenated blood makes its way up to the brain and the sensory organs. When inverting, the pressure is reversed. Some research indicates the presence of internal mechanisms that sense the increase in blood and slow the flow, thus reducing both blood pressure and heart rate.

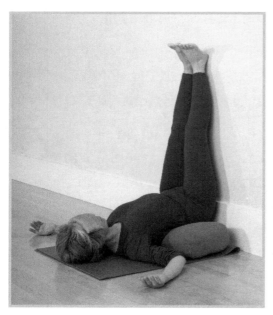

Supported Legs Up the Wall Pose, **Viparita Karani.** *Krishna Raman, M.D., states that in* **Viparita Karani,** *"The blood flow collects in the pelvis and this spills over like a waterfall to the heart, flushing open the cardiac vessels."*

Studies have shown that even at the age
of 85 or 90, individuals can be trained to a level of
physical fitness [equal to] that of a young person.
This is essentially practice and careful understanding
of the subject. The human body can achieve much;
we must know the intricate details and
methods of how to do so.

Krishna Raman, M.D.,
Yoga and Medical Science

Lying Back Over a Backbender
(*Viparita Dandasana* on a Backbender)

The Backbender is a whale-shaped object that stretches the shoulders and the spine and opens the heart/chest area. The stronger supported backbends, such as Lying Back Over a Backbender or Chair, have a powerful physiological effect on the nervous system, glands, and organs. You can feel the massage of your inner organs during a long stay in these poses. The chest expands, opening the heart center.

When your muscles are too tight or weak, or you are afraid of putting your body in positions or shapes that it has not been in for many years, props are a way of removing the obstacles between you and a pose that seems out of reach. The Back-bender supports and lengthens your spine, stretches your arms and shoulders, opens your rib cage and lungs, and counteracts the rounding of the upper back, deepens your breathing, and stretches the groin, abdomen, and front of the thighs.

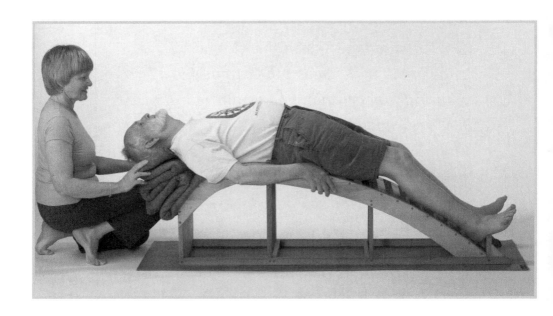

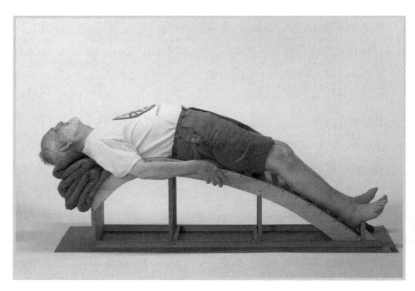

An eighty-year-old beginner on the backbender, his neck and head supported.

Lying Back Over a Chair—Inverted Staff Pose
(*Viparita Dandasana* on a Chair)

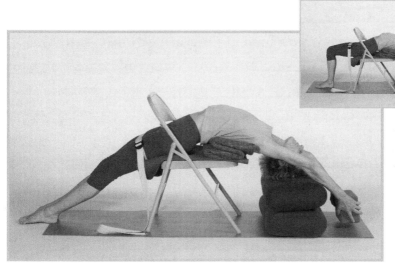

Inverted Staff Posture on the chair, variation, knees bent.

Inverted Staff Posture, **Viparita Dandasana,** *on the chair. Two bolsters under the head, a strap around the thighs, legs straight, feet flat on floor, arms overhead, hands stretching toward the blocks.*

- Place a sturdy chair (a yoga folding chair is best) about two feet away from a wall. The exact distance depends on your leg length: far enough so that when you straighten your legs you can place your toes or entire foot on the wall, as illustrated.

- Place a folded sticky mat or blanket over the front edge of the seat.

- Sit backward on the chair, facing the wall, with your legs through the chair. Scoot your bottom toward the wall in front of you so that when you lean back your head and neck extend past the chair seat, and your shoulder blades drape over the edge of the seat.

- Hold onto the sides of the chair as you slowly arch backward. If you have a long upper body and your shoulder blades do not drape over the chair seat, scoot your bottom farther toward the back edge of the seat (toward the wall in front of you).

- Take your feet toward the wall, and as you straighten your legs, press your feet into the wall.

- If you are a beginner or if you feel any discomfort in your back, place your feet higher up against the wall or on a bolster or other height, so that your feet are level with your pelvis.

- Beginners can stay in the pose for about thirty seconds to one minute. Experienced practitioners can increase the length of time gradually and benefit greatly from a long stay in this pose.

- To come out, bend your knees, place your feet on the floor close to the chair, hold onto the back of the chair and carefully come up, lifting the chest. It is restful to gently lean forward over the back of the chair. Carefully come out of the chair. Rest in Child's Pose.

Caution: *Learn this pose under the guidance of an experienced teacher. If you have back or neck problems, your teacher can show you how to place props to support your head, neck, and back in this pose, as illustrated.*

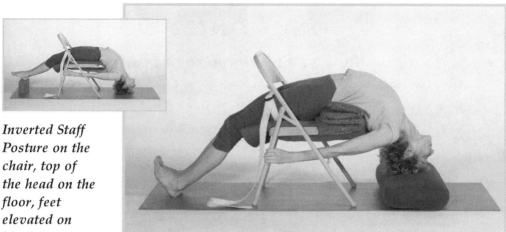

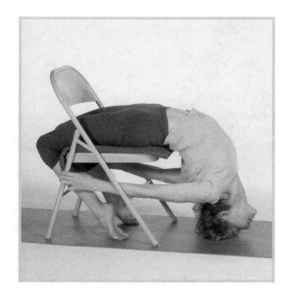

Inverted Staff Posture on the chair, top of the head on the floor, feet elevated on block, arms inside front rungs of chair.

Inverted Staff Posture on the chair, one bolster under the head, strap around thighs, legs straight, heels pressing down but feet off floor, arms inside front rungs of chair.

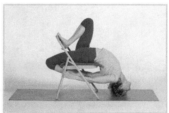

Little Thunderbolt Pose in the chair, variation, prepare to lift one leg.

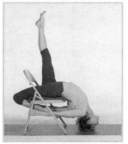

*Little Thunderbolt Pose, **Laghu Vajrasana,** in the chair.*

Little Thunderbolt Pose with one leg up, variation in the chair.

TONI MONTEZ

Looking Back at Eighty on Yoga in My Life

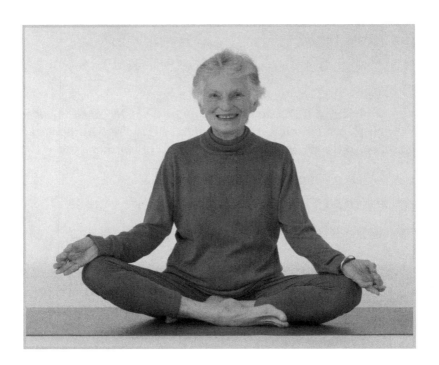

*T*oni Montez was born on March 28, 1927. She was on the staff of the Iyengar Yoga Institute of San Francisco for many years and was one of my first teachers. She studied with B. K. S. Iyengar in India and was instrumental in bringing master teachers, such as Dona Holleman, to the United States. Toni's area of expertise includes relaxation and stress reduction. I asked Toni to share her thoughts on life and yoga.

We were living in Australia for two years when I was first able to enter a yoga class. I was in my early forties and thought it was time for some regular exercise. Jogging or tennis did not appeal to me, but yoga seemed gentle, relatively easy, and the poses quite lovely. Soon after starting classes, I began experiencing changes that I had not anticipated. I had a new sense of myself, a confidence and a calmness that were truly different for me. Although I had no religious beliefs, I suddenly found a birth of spiritual philosophy that was truly startling.

These transformations brought about a strong desire to share with others what I had learned. After returning from Australia, I started studying and teaching, and a whole new world opened up for me. It was exciting. I enjoyed the teaching, and it went well.

Twenty years later my son, Kim, died suddenly and unexpectedly at the age of thirty-five. He was born with a hole in his heart and had gone through open-heart surgery as a child. He and I were close, and his passing was the most difficult period of my life. We had done a great deal of traveling together, and I had learned a lot from him.

My good friend Dona Holleman told me to just practice my asanas, but I felt I couldn't do that because they helped me mask my feelings. I didn't want to overcome my grief. I wanted to experience it fully. Doing yoga works differently with different people, but I knew that my emotions would not be allowed their fullness if I did too much yoga practice.

In 2001, I was told that I had early-stage rectal cancer. I had relatively minor surgery to remove the cancer. Recovery was fairly fast, and the six weeks of radiation that followed were without problems. Soon after the radiation I left for South America with Dona to enjoy yoga courses and recreation.

Upon my return from South America, I learned that the cancer had returned and required a much more invasive surgery and the loss of my rectum. I had one more major abdominal surgery that year that was unrelated to the cancer. The series of surgeries removed or weakened many muscles and caused considerable difficulties.

Although there are quite a few yoga poses that I can no longer do, I am healthy and active and feel that yoga helped my body and psyche through the process of surgery and recovery. While teaching yoga, I had studied many relaxation techniques and had taught one that I thought was the most effective. This is one thing that I never stopped doing, and it has helped me through all my difficult situations.

At eighty, I'm still busily clearing areas of my large yard, which is a never-ending project and heavy work. I also walk my dog twice a day. During these activities, I experience a different element of yoga. Both were healing for me during the grieving process.

My practice is now comfortable and sometimes difficult. I do a shoulderstand and some backbending poses. Backbends are important to stimulate the adrenals after menopause. Several years ago I added some weights for leg and hip strengthening. Osteoporosis was something that yoga, alone, could not solve for me, and it is important to realize that yoga doesn't do everything. Walking and other strengthening activities are also important.

There is no question that yoga has altered my life in many beneficial ways. It has helped make me strong and able to absorb life more philosophically. It has opened new avenues and given me the courage to follow them. It has kept me feeling youthful, healthy, and energetic. It has encouraged me to enjoy life and to be ever thankful for all that life has to offer.

CHAPTER 9

Yoga for
Parkinson's Disease

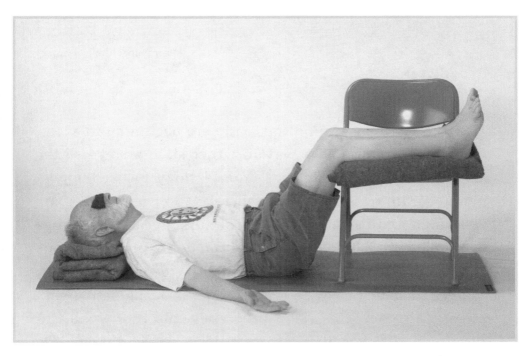

Deep Relaxation Pose (Corpse Pose), **Savasana,** *with the lower legs on a chair, an eye bag over the eyes, and a folded blanket under the head. This stress-reducing position is very relaxing for the whole body, especially the lower back.*

If you have Parkinson's disease,
it's important to recognize that the condition
is one that demands adaptation, not despair.
Learning to pace yourself, prioritize goals and make
timely use of allied health strategies to enhance
your physical, intellectual and emotional well-being
can make all the difference in how you enjoy
life and maintain your independence.

Paul Nausieda, M.D.,
movement disorders specialist,
Aurora Sinai Medical Center

Researchers around the world are beginning to examine exercise as a way to either slow or reverse the effects of Parkinson's. Yoga's slow, focused movements, breathing awareness, and relaxation techniques are well suited for this purpose. Many of the suggestions for yoga for people with Parkinson's disease can be adapted to anyone who has problems with balance and movement in daily life.

Parkinson's disease (PD) is defined as a "degenerative neurological disorder." It is a slow progressive disorder of the central nervous system that was first described in 1817 by Dr. James Parkinson.

Symptoms range from shaking, tremors, and muscle rigidity to impaired balance and loss of fine motor skills. These symptoms make life increasingly difficult. Other characteristics of PD include absence of facial expression, shuffling of feet when walking, difficulty breathing and swallowing, dizziness, and a forward stooping posture. The changes in posture and movement impair balance and increase the tendency to fall. The types of symptoms present and the rate at which this disease progresses vary greatly from person to person.

Globally, it is estimated that 6.3 million people have PD. In the United States alone an estimated 1.5 million people have it, and 60,000 new cases are diagnosed each year.

PD typically affects older adults, but—as the world learned when the actor Michael J. Fox was diagnosed with PD at age 29—it also affects younger people. The average age of onset is the early sixties, and it affects approximately 10 percent of people over age seventy-five.

In simple terms, PD is the result of a deficiency of dopamine, which is a chemical substance in the brain. Dopamine allows us to move smoothly and normally.

It was phenomenal to see students
with noticeable tremors relax in Savasana.
All the students experienced a quieting
of their tremors, and in some cases students were
tremor free by the end of Savasana.

A teacher describing students at a
Yoga for Parkinson's workshop

PD is difficult to diagnose because there are no specific x-rays or blood tests to determine its presence. It can be diagnosed only through observation and thorough examination.

Current treatment is aimed at managing and reducing symptoms and keeping people as healthy, active, and independent as possible. Treatment can include medication, surgery, and healthy lifestyle changes, including nutrition, massage, yoga, and other forms of low-impact exercise.

As in many areas of medicine, patients, physicians, and other practitioners are looking outside traditional therapies to find ways to treat various aspects of PD and the side effects of treatment. Modern medications and surgical therapies for PD have made tremendous advances in improving the quality and length of life. Many sources of information on alternative and complementary treatments for PD, are available, some of which are listed in Appendix C.

While yoga cannot cure PD, it can help manage and reduce symptoms by improving breathing habits, muscle strength, flexibility, balance, body mechanics, and the ability to initiate movement.

Yoga for Parkinson's

Studies have shown yoga to be one of the most beneficial alternative therapies for people with PD. The largest PD research center in the United States is located in Milwaukee, Wisconsin. In 2003, the Milwaukee Yoga Center began offering Yoga for Parkinson's workshops and classes, taught by Iyengar yoga teachers and their assistants. Instructors included Chris Saudek, a senior Iyengar teacher who is also a physical therapist with firsthand experience with yoga for PD patients.

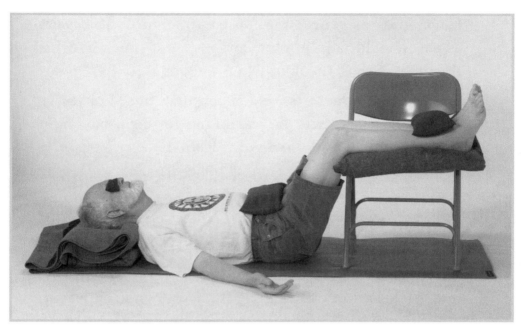

Deep Relaxation Pose (Corpse Pose), **Savasana.** *The addition of a sandbag across pelvis and shins helps the body to relax.*

Under the watchful eyes of teachers and assistants in these workshops, students with PD and their caregivers are taught a series of standing poses to improve their motor skills, balance, and range of motion, and they are supported in lying-down poses that decrease stress and promote relaxation.

Teaching People with Parkinson's Disease

In her writings about her experience teaching people with PD, yoga teacher Jeanette Macturk, now in her eighties, gives the following advice to teachers:

- Have students concentrate on breath control *(pranayama)* as this should help in moments of panic—such as when their feet stick to the floor when walking.

- Encourage students to remember that the slowness of their movements may be frustrating to them, but this is purely physical, and the mind will still be very alert.

- PD itself does not necessarily weaken the muscles. This is usually caused by lack of movement as individuals withdraw into themselves, so exercise is good. Encourage daily practice—but not enough to cause fatigue.

- Do not be discouraged if your group is small. Helping even one single Parkinson's sufferer is a worthwhile endeavor.

Yoga for People with Parkinson's Disease

The rigidity of muscles and postural changes that are associated with PD respond well to regular yoga practice. B. K. S. Iyengar notes in *Yoga: The Path to Holistic Health* that people with PD may find it helpful to stand facing a wall, with the palms placed on it, when standing in Mountain Pose, *Tadasana*. Mountain Pose and the other standing poses teach the art of standing correctly with the weight balanced perfectly on both legs and both feet and with the head, neck, and spine in a straight line. Mountain Pose counters the degenerative effects of aging on the spine, legs, and feet and helps us to establish a sense of being steady on our feet.

Progress with the Parkinson's Project

All who have participated in the Parkinson's project agree that it has been an amazing experience. The spirit of the Parkinson's patients has touched all the instructors and assistants. Regardless of the stage of disease and the difficulties the patients had in walking, all the Parkinson's students were game enough to venture out in sometimes bitter cold Wisconsin weather and try something new in an unfamiliar place with unknown teachers, trusting that Iyengar yoga could help alleviate some of the symptoms of their disease. Despite their age (many in their seventies and eighties) and illness, they had not given up. Every student put out great amounts of physical and mental effort and seemed to really enjoy the challenge of the activity and the camaraderie. Many of the students surprised themselves (and at times the staff!) on what they could do and how much better they felt. Besides increased flexibility and balance, there was also a noticeable increase in self-confidence among the students. After several classes, students who were able would come in to the studio and set up props for themselves and the rest of their classmates. With each class they became more knowledgeable and self-sufficient.

Chris Saudek, Director, The Yoga Place,
La Crosse, Wisconsin

Years ago when I helped care for elderly people with PD, I mainly helped with activities of daily living (ADLs). ADLs include eating, going to the toilet, getting dressed, taking a bath or shower, and walking or moving about in general to accomplish these tasks. Some symptoms of PD (tremor, stiffness, slow movement, and balance problems) may worsen over time and can make it more difficult to do these daily life tasks that are essential for independent living.

A holistic program for those with PD will include instruction in body mechanics, walking, moving around, preventing falls, getting down to and back up from the floor—all of which should be part of a regular yoga class for older students. Using correct body mechanics helps to protect the joints from injury and reduces the risk of falls and other accidents.

Teachers can emphasize the importance of incorporating into daily life the posture and balance awareness learned in class. Walking, sitting in and getting out of a chair, and lying on a floor and getting back up are all occasions for practicing such awareness.

When falls happen, the person is often alone. This can be a frightening experience, and the more panic sets in, the less likely a person will be able to get back up by himself or herself.

When I worked as a home healthcare provider, on several occasions I arrived to find my patient on the floor. Sometimes he or she had been waiting for me for several hours. Falling while home alone is a significant danger for people with PD and for older people in general. It is a leading reason why people lose their independence and are transitioned into a nursing home.

Getting Down to and Up from the Floor: Essential for Independent Living

In our modern world, where sitting and lying on the floor are often not part of daily life, many people lose the ability as they grow older to easily get down to and up from the floor. One of the great perks of going to a yoga class regularly is that in the course of a typical class you will sit, kneel, and lie on the floor both on your back and on your stomach. Each time you get up from the floor you are strengthening the arm, leg, back, and abdominal muscles needed to ensure that you maintain this essential skill for safe, independent living.

The fear of falling can be considerably lessened by experimenting with techniques for lowering one's body to the floor and getting up again (see Chapter 10). When people with PD and, in general, older people are taught in a yoga class how to get down to and up from the floor, they are more likely to be able to get back up on their own if they fall.

By practicing mindful movements in class, students with PD learn to pause, take some deep breaths, relax, and more calmly think their way through a situation. By practicing getting up and down in class, they are more apt to get up calmly on their own.

Practicing yoga postures helps students improve balance, flexibility, joint range of motion, and body awareness. Since rigidity of the muscles is common for those with PD, a gentle yoga practice allows them to move and explore their bodies while becoming aware of its needs.

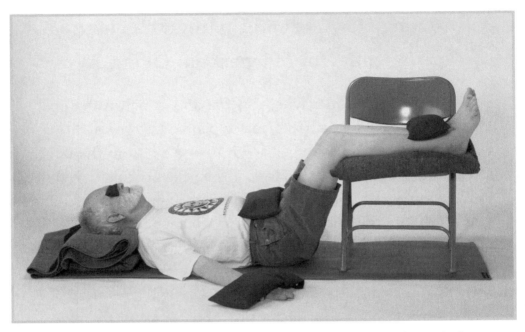

Here Deep Relaxation Pose is practiced with additional weight on the lower arms and hands to allow the body to access even deeper levels of relaxation.

Stress and Parkinson's Disease

As with many other chronic diseases, PD symptoms may increase under stress, and the characteristic tremor gets worse with stress and fatigue. Stressful events can also accelerate the progression of the disease. Yoga helps those with PD to cope with stress, depression, insomnia, and other problems associated with medical procedures.

In addition, yoga may help decrease pain and the need for pain medication; decrease side effects and complications of medical procedures; shorten hospital stays and the time it takes to recover; strengthen the immune system; and enhance the ability to heal. All these benefits help to improve self-confidence and one's outlook on life.

Yoga students with PD report that meditation—consciously regulating their breath, calming and quieting the mind—can help them control their tremors. When a tremor starts, a common reaction is to become upset or self-conscious, which tends to exacerbate the condition. If instead of reacting to a tremor the person with PD begins to inhale and exhale calmly and bring the mind into a meditative state, the nervous system calms and the tremor stops.

Note: *The International Association of Yoga Therapists provides a comprehensive listing of resources on yoga and Parkinson's disease. For more information, see Appendix C.*

JANICE FREEMAN-BELL

Yoga for Parkinson's Disease—Exploration and Acceptance

*J*anice Freeman-Bell is a Registered Yoga Teacher and Certified Senior Fitness Instructor who has taught older students for over twenty years. She has studied with many of the most influential teachers in the world, which keeps her classes for seniors lively, fun, and fresh! Janice is the mother of three children and four grandchildren. Her other love is music, and she is skilled at leading groups in songs, musical meditations, and chants at yoga retreats. She has produced a beautiful CD, One Thousand Cranes.

I've been practicing yoga since my mid-twenties. My first yoga teacher was in her seventies and inspired me with her balance and flexibility. She performed the most difficult poses with such gentle grace that I wanted to be just like her! Unfortunately, I was not a disciplined student and just danced around the edges of yoga for several years. In my early fifties and recovering from divorce, I returned to yoga in a dedicated way.

I have worked in senior fitness programs for over twenty years as an adult education teacher with city schools and currently with a university-sponsored program for seniors. Most of our students had no prior exposure to yoga and a very gentle asana program was presented to them with dynamic results. These are busy, active seniors! They have found that regular yoga classes keep them "de-stressed," flexible, strong, and balanced.

One of my yoga students has Parkinson's disease and has experienced such well-being with yoga that our university recently conducted an eight-week pilot study on the benefits of yoga for people with Parkinson's disease. The class was developed with professionals in older adult fitness, yoga instructors, and physical therapists.

Seven men and three women participated in the program. Some of the students also practiced at home during the week. Everyone showed physical and mental improvement. Two physical therapists and five interns assisted me and were impressed with the results. The results were so positive that we are in the process of putting together a larger, longer study.

As a certified yoga teacher, I knew that we were dealing with energy and intention—not simply stretching exercises! Yoga addresses the mental, emotional, and spiritual areas that help improve quality of life and help people cope. We added Yoga for Parkinson's to our yoga curriculum as a result of our pilot research program.

My personal yoga practice is one of exploration and acceptance—especially now in my sixties. I love my flexible hamstrings, strong arms, and stamina. Some poses work for me, while others don't—and I am okay with it.

What is most important to me, however, is the spiritual aspect of my life and how yoga has brought a quietness to it. Long meditations with contemplative prayer and chanting are a regular part of my day. I feel that these are certainly my wisdom years, and I intend to bask in that light and continue to share the vision of yoga—that indeed yoga is for everyone!

Note: *For more information about the pilot Yoga Program for People with Parkinson's, contact Janice Freeman-Bell at Janicefb@surewest.net.*

ALEXANDRA (SANDRA) PLEASANTS
Teaching Yoga to People with Parkinson's Disease

*S*andra Pleasants is a senior Iyengar yoga teacher who resides and teaches in Virginia. She offers the following advice regarding teaching students with Parkinson's disease.

I have taught several courses of ten weeks' duration to students with Parkinson's who have said that the class gave them confidence, improved their balance, and in general made them feel better.

The first thing I taught these students was how to get up and down from the floor using a chair as an aid. This is good practice for people who tend to fall, and it is good exercise if you repeat it several times.

Once we were down on the floor, we did what I call "finger and toe weaving," as many of the students suffered from neuropathy in their feet. We often laughed about ending up with the same number of fingers and toes.

We did some modified standing poses with emphasis on standing up tall, as in *Tadasana* (Mountain Pose). For many of the students balance is an issue, so we often used the wall or a chair as a prop.

The students tired easily, so the classes were only one hour. Their favorite part of the class was Supported Bound-Angle Pose, *Supta Baddha Konasana*. At the end of class, they always asked for more time in this pose. It was their deep relaxation.

I learned from the participants how to teach them. I don't know how well it would work to integrate students with Parkinson's into a regular class, but some of them were in good physical shape and could probably participate in a gentle yoga class.

CHAPTER 10

The Art of Teaching Seniors

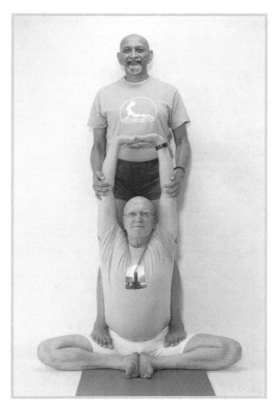

Bound-Angle Pose. Master yoga teacher Ramanand Patel anchors the legs of his student and helps him stretch upward. This advanced adjustment must be learned from an expert instructor. Do not try this on your own!

*The age group that needs the most
health support (55 plus) is either unfamiliar
with yoga's health benefits, or is preconditioned to
seek only medical solutions offered by traditional medical
treatment modalities, such as drugs and surgery.
Yoga, taught by professionals who are skilled in
teaching seniors, could greatly reduce the rapidly
rising costs of senior medical care, the costs of
institutionalization, the use of prescription medicine,
as well as other health related medical services.*

Frank and Serpil Iszak,
founders, Silver Age Yoga Community
Outreach, silverageyoga.org

T his chapter is devoted to the art of teaching seniors—
those who should be highly esteemed, as they are in
the upper grades of the school of life. Many of the
suggestions here will also be helpful for older beginners practicing at home.

In the world of yoga, a senior teacher is one who has
studied for years with master teachers and has achieved an
advanced level of proficiency. These teachers are not necessarily advanced in years. However, a teacher over age fifty-five
can also be referred to as *senior* simply by virtue of being older.

Many of us tend to shy away from the association of the
word *senior* with antiquated notions about aging. However, if
we associate it with the idea of seniority and with wisdom,

then maybe we won't mind being called a *senior citizen*.

In over thirty years of teaching yoga, I've learned that students of all ages, older just as much as younger, can benefit from the same vital weight-bearing postures. The main adjustment necessary for teaching older beginners is to proceed at a slower pace with the support of plenty of props! This helps to ensure safety, conserves energy, and is more harmonious with the later stage of life.

Teaching any class that is geared to a special segment of the population starts with understanding the needs and challenges of the people in that group—whether it is yoga for kids, athletes, or women who are pregnant or approaching menopause.

However, as with any age group, the differences among older individuals defy stereotype or attempts at defining what is typical. As my teacher Toni Montez pointed out, "There's no general rule, except that you're teaching people, not yoga. You treat people individually, and everyone's going to be different."

The most successful senior Yoga classes
are those where the people feel respected and inspired
to explore. Don't talk down to them. Bring lightness in
how you speak to them and the tone of your voice.
Bring it to a level where you are communicating to them
at a more personal, informal level. Be one of them.

Frank Iszak, age 75, yoga teacher and
founder of Silver Age Yoga

Advice for Teaching Seniors

An essential element in the education of any teacher who is training to work with older people is to observe and interact with them in their day-to-day environments. Spend time visiting and helping older family members, neighbors, and acquaintances in their homes. Before teaching your first class, visit and observe in senior centers and in assisted living facilities.

For older students, the motivation to do yoga is not just to play a better game of tennis or look better or lower blood pressure. Many come to their first class when they begin to realize that everyday activities are becoming difficult. They need the practice of yoga to help them remain mobile and to regain their ability to function well. Otherwise, they may become increasingly incapacitated.

Many older practitioners, especially those with years of experience, are aware of their bodies and are not apt to hurt themselves. However, a great many older beginners come to yoga extremely stiff and with parts of their bodies virtually immobilized.

Simple movements younger people take for granted, such as placing hands flat on a floor or a wall, can become almost impossible for older students. Over time, long-standing physical problems become magnified, and the body freezes into the shape of habitual postures. Older students often accept these limitations as an inevitable part of aging, but as they practice the yoga postures, their awareness and sensitivity return.

Senior Psychology

Understanding my life in the framework
of the seasons allows me to see the value in each phase.
As we get older, it can be easy to give in to hopelessness
as we finally recognize our mortality. But when we
understand that our afternoon and sunset years
have a value and a purpose all their own, we gain a
new appreciation for these years. Suddenly we
desire to live them for all they're worth!

Lilias Folan,
Lilias! Yoga Gets Better with Age

A teacher must be sensitive to the energy levels and emotional conditions of their students. The class atmosphere should be both physically and spiritually uplifting so it doesn't add additional stress to a student's psyche.

When I look around at my group of seniors, I am aware that many are going through very difficult periods in their lives. Often someone in the class is grieving, has little energy, or is on medication for depression. Some are coping not only with their own health issues, but also with a spouse with Alzheimer's or another disease. The yoga class may be one of the rare hours in the week that they do something for themselves.

The social aspect of the class is very important. There are many ways that a teacher can incorporate the students' need to socialize and interact with like-minded people in a way that is not disruptive to the class. Allow for time before and after class for people to interact with one another. If you teach in a location where people cannot comfortably socialize before and after class, your students will end up chatting in the parking lot or on the sidewalk. The yoga class can serve as a tremendous support system for all ages, but especially the elderly.

Part of learning how to teach older people is to deepen our understanding of the last years of life. Society's attitudes toward aging and death are gradually changing, but many of us are not familiar with what happens in this stage of life. We see shooting and violent death on TV and elsewhere, but many of us have little or no firsthand acquaintance with the process of dying of old age or disease. With that experience comes a whole new attitude.

The spiritual life includes facing death. As yoga teachers, we must face this in ourselves and teach with that awareness. Many opportunities to openly discuss death and dying present themselves naturally in the course of teaching seniors. Teachers must be sensitive to these occasions and not deny or avoid them.

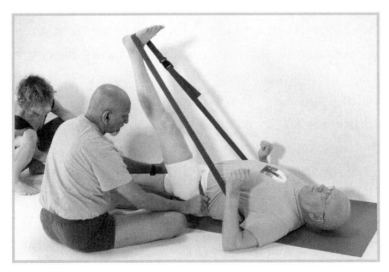

Lying-Down Big Toe Pose as practiced with a long yoga strap around each foot.

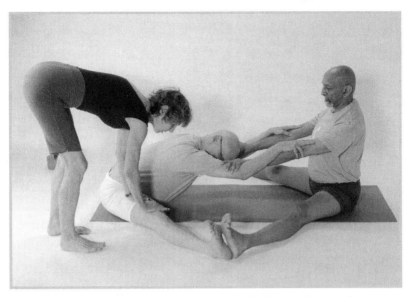

Seated Wide-Angle Pose. Two teachers are helping the student to anchor and align his pelvis and legs so that he can elongate his upper body to the maximum.

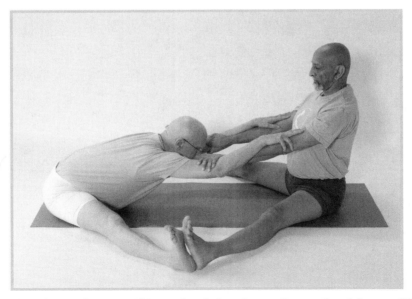

Seated Wide-Angle Pose. The teacher helps the student to bend forward from the pelvis.

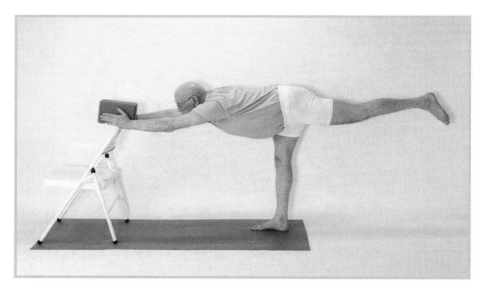

Warrior III Pose, **Virabhadrasana III,** *practiced with the support of a chair. Standing poses can first be practiced lying down on the floor. Turn this page upside down to see how the pose looks when it is practiced on your back.*

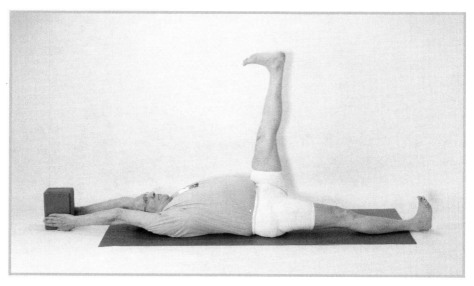

Warrior III Pose preparation, lying down. Turn this page upside down to see how this pose looks from a standing position.

Tips for Teaching Older Students

Don't treat me like an old lady!

An older student speaking to her teacher

• A group dynamic is at work in all classes, especially in older groups. While yoga is noncompetitive, the group dynamic strongly influences the results of the individual and the class as a whole. The more that older people see their peers practicing more challenging poses, the more they will expect of themselves.

• Be ever alert that you do not impose your own myths about aging on your students. It continues to be a revelation to me to witness the extent of the progress made by my older students.

• As people grow older, they often feel unsteady on their feet. Loss of hearing, eyesight, strength, and flexibility and the side effects of medication all affect balance and coordination. The yoga standing poses reestablish our connection to Planet Earth. Students develop a sense of groundedness, stability, and balance. Mountain Pose, *Tadasana*, and other standing poses can help seniors regain confidence in standing on their own two feet!

• Start with standing poses with the back of the body against a wall or other support, with a chair available for the lower hand. If you have plenty of chairs and plenty of space, put one chair on either side.

- When space is unavailable for the whole back of the body to be against a wall, have students practice standing poses with the back foot anchored against the baseboard. You can divide the class in half and have more experienced students in the center of the room. The more experienced students will serve as visual role models for the beginners, who can practice the same poses with the support of a wall or table.

- Students can also hold onto the upper wall rope (when available) with the upper hand and place the lower hand on a chair for additional support. With this level of support, all my older students—even octogenarians taking their first-ever yoga class—safely practice all the basic standing poses, including poses that require balancing on one leg.

- In a class of students with many physical problems, start with simple lying-down poses and gradually work up to standing postures. The firm, even surface of the floor, like the wall, is a great teacher. Teach Mountain Pose, *Tadasana*, both lying down and standing upright against a wall. Before students lie down, be sure they have the props they need within reach.

- The firm, level surface of the floor helps to teach good body alignment, but those who find it uncomfortable may need an extra mat or blanket under the back and head. Have students practice resting their bodies as evenly on the floor as possible for at least ten minutes every day.

- Be sure students do not hyperextend their necks in any pose. When students are lying down, make sure that the curve at the back of the neck is not extreme. The head should not be tilted back, and the forehead should not be lower than the chin. Hyperextension of the back of the neck can reduce blood flow to the brain, which can cause fainting or even a stroke. Place a folded blanket, block, or book under the head to bring the forehead level or slightly higher than the chin.

- Avoid poses that bear weight directly on the neck. Older people often have weak, porous vertebrae, vulnerable to injury. Older people should learn weight-bearing inverted poses such as Headstand and Shoulderstand under the guidance of an experienced instructor, preferably in a private lesson or small group class where the teacher works with students individually.

- When bending forward from a standing or seated position, have students move from the hip joint with the upper body in one unit, the spine elongated so that they are creating space in their bodies and not collapsing the chest, lungs, or spine. If the muscles at the back of the thighs (hamstrings) are tight, it is difficult to bend forward without rounding and consequently compressing the back—especially the thoracic spine, which is the area most at risk for fracture. Walls, chairs, and other props are invaluable for learning how to lengthen the spine and create space between the vertebrae.

- Avoid any movement that reinforces a rounded back (kyphosis) or hunched, collapsed positions that exacerbate poor posture. All movements in which the upper body is hunched can intensify the forces that result in vertebral crush fractures (one of the reasons older people lose height). Have students practice Standing Forward Bend Poses with their hands on a wall, chair, desk, table, or counter. Yoga's seated poses should be practiced with at least two firmly folded blankets under the buttocks to help maintain the integrity of the spinal column. It is critical that older students understand the principle of bending forward from the hip joints and not from the lower back.

• The pace of the class is extremely important. A slower pace makes it possible for older people to do the postures safely and to deeply connect the mind, body, and breath. Instructions must be clear and easy to follow and are usually better understood if they are both visual and verbal.

• Teach (and practice) at least one inverted pose. Remind students that inversions counteract the aging process by reversing the gravitational pull on the internal organs and improving blood flow returning to the heart. Teaching older students how to invert safely is one of the greatest gifts of yoga.

• Many older people have some level of hearing loss. If a student does not respond to directions, it may be because he or she cannot hear you or, in some cases, clearly see you. Remember to speak loudly and clearly. Make a point to stand near students who have difficulty hearing. My students with hearing aids remind me that while a hearing aid can make sounds louder, it doesn't necessarily make them clearer. Be aware that hearing aids can "ring" if your hands come too close to the student's ears when you are adjusting his or her neck and head in *Savasana* or other poses.

- Encourage students to attend class on a regular basis and to practice the poses at home. Emphasize the benefits of each posture.

The Art of Getting Down to and Up from the Floor

When one of my editors on the home front read this section of the manuscript she said, "How hard can it be to get on the floor—you don't need to explain this, do you?" I proceeded to explain that people who are not in the habit of getting down to the floor in daily life gradually lose the ability to do so. I even demonstrated how people are sometimes afraid they will fall on their knees the first time they lower themselves to the ground. Getting down and up is especially difficult for heavier people with weak quadriceps and knee and hip problems.

My editor was still incredulous. She said, "Well, maybe when someone is eighty or ninety. But not younger." I reminded her that we don't lose the ability to do something overnight. We are a car–couch culture! Gardening, yoga, and getting on the floor with grandchildren are all good antidotes to sitting in cars and furniture. Losing the neuromuscular pathway for getting down to and up from the floor is the end result of many years of not sitting or lying on the floor.

My students who are in their eighties and nineties get up from and down to the floor with relative ease several times during the course of a typical class. But very often, when they bring a friend or family member of similar age to class, I notice them helping their guest to and from the floor. Their guest might even balk at the idea and end up sitting in a chair. When someone tells me "I'll just sit in a chair instead of going on the floor," with rare exceptions I explain that regaining the ability to sit and lie on the floor is one of the most important parts of their first lessons.

When newcomers see other people their age or older getting down to and up from the floor, it often helps give them confidence that they can do it too. Sometimes that is all that is needed to overcome psychological barriers.

Students unsure about getting on the floor unassisted generally find it helpful to lower and raise themselves up with the help of a sturdy chair placed on a yoga sticky mat and braced securely against a wall—a corner wall, if available, is even better.

Be absolutely sure to position the chair so that it will not slip or collapse. If necessary, the chair can be made more secure by placing several ten-pound yoga sandbags near the back of the chair seat or the rung between the back legs of the chair. If there is any doubt about the stability of the chair, the teacher or helper can secure the chair with his or her own weight so that the student does not have to worry about the chair moving or collapsing.

A folded blanket on top of a sticky mat near the chair seat makes kneeling less painful. If wall ropes are available, position the chair near the ropes so that the student can use the ropes and the chair.

Safety is my first concern when assessing the strength, flexibility, and coordination of a new student. I stand nearby to make sure the student does not fall, and I offer assistance as needed.

If I see that the student is having a lot of difficulty I may suggest, "Try turning to your other side," or "See which side, which arm, which leg is stronger."

I assure students that it's fine to take all the time they need to figure out how to get up and down. In some instances, it may take several minutes. Students may even need to rest before attempting to get up or down again. As with anything else, with practice it gets easier.

I constantly remind my older students to sit on the floor every day, the way children do. I remind them to descend to the floor and get back up at least twice a day, preferably more often. At home they can practice near a couch. In our chair-oriented culture, where hips and leg muscles are often very stiff, many people have difficulty lowering their bottoms to their heels.

Note: *When the neuromuscular pathways for getting up and down are used regularly, it is easier to recover if, by chance, you should slip and fall.*

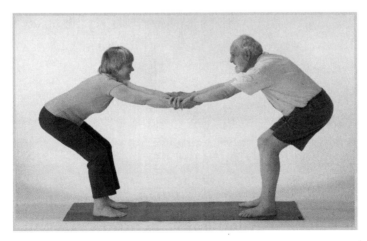

The teacher helps the student to balance while practicing Chair Pose. This pose helps students lower themselves to the floor.

Moving to and from the Floor:
Step-by-Step Hints for Students

• Have someone nearby to assist you if necessary.

• Stand next to a sturdy chair or other piece of furniture near a wall. If your balance is very unstable or leg muscles are very weak, try standing between two chairs or other stable supports that you can hold or use as a brace. From standing, holding onto the support as needed, step forward and begin to lower your knees to the floor.

• Kneeling on one or both knees, lower your bottom toward your heels. Holding the chair with one hand, with the other hand on the floor, is helpful as you try sitting to the side of your feet. Use your arms to lower yourself to the floor.

• To stand up, reverse this process. Or try another way. In the process of trying you will find a way to get back up that works for you.

• With daily practice your muscles will strengthen and the movement will become easier.

• I cannot overemphasize the importance of maintaining the ability to get up and down from the floor. Practicing this will also make it easier to get up from chairs and other places, even if the seat is low.

Note: *Yoga wall ropes, described in Chapter 4, are extremely useful for people with balance problems and difficulty getting down to and up from the floor. Wall ropes can be purchased for home use (see Appendix C).*

Note: *See Chapter 11 for sequences of poses that I use regularly in my senior classes. These same sequences can be practiced at home.*

*My practice has changed, particularly
over the past few years, now that I'm in my sixties.
Yoga made me strong in spirit and body. It kept me whole
through cancer and its awful treatments. It calmed
my mind through turmoil, losses, and grieving.
It made me feel physically powerful.
Now, as I get older, I am sometimes frustrated
that my body won't cooperate as it used to. So I am
very happy to be in class with Suza and other people
who are going through the same issues and help
me enjoy the delicious asanas that we practice.
We accept and embrace our bodies as they are, regardless
of age, which is what yoga has taught me.*

Catherine Meek, yoga student

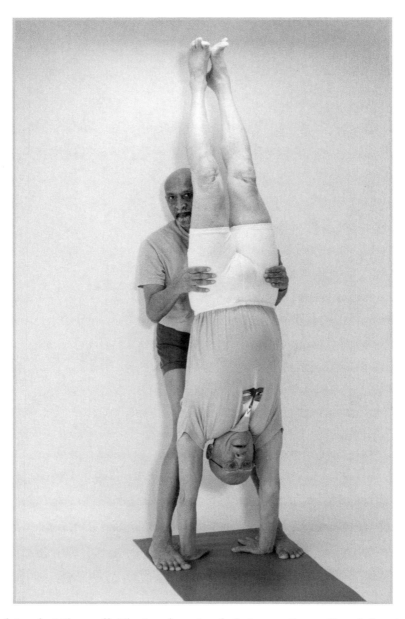

Handstand at the wall. The teacher stands between the wall and the student to help him balance and extend upward.

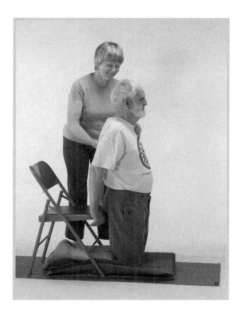

Camel Pose with a chair. The teacher encourages the student to open his chest.

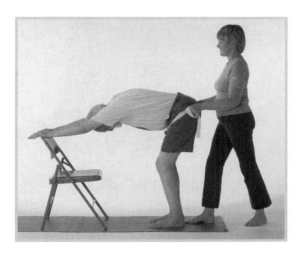

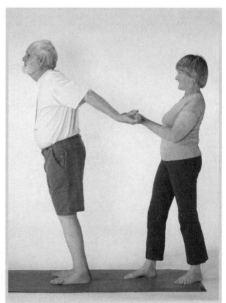

The teacher helps the student to stretch the hips back to lengthen the spine.

The teacher helps the student to stretch his shoulders in Mountain Pose.

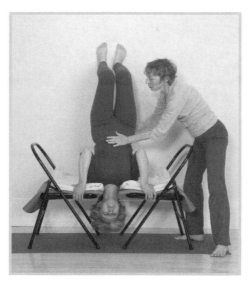

Headstand with two chairs and a wall. The teacher makes sure the student is practicing the pose safely.

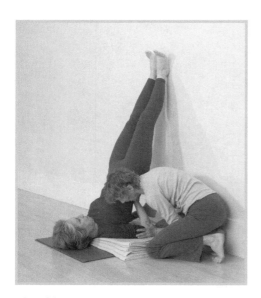

Shoulderstand at the Wall. The teacher helps the student to support her back.

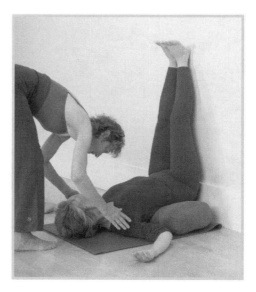

*Supported Legs Up the Wall Pose, **Viparita Karani**. The teacher adjusts the student's shoulders and checks that the neck is comfortable.*

LEIGH MILNE

Full Circle—Reflections on Teaching Yoga to Seniors

*When young, yoga develops our outer strength
and as we age, yoga develops our inner strength.
Yoga looks after us throughout our life.*

Leigh Milne

*L*eigh Milne is a certified Iyengar yoga teacher and a registered yoga teacher. She has studied with the Iyengars on several occasions at the Ramamani Memorial Yoga Institute in Pune, India. She enjoys teaching older adults. With help from a grant funded by the Central Vermont Council on Aging, she authored a study on the benefits of yoga for seniors (see Appendix C.)

When my longtime yoga teacher, Shirley Davenport-French, turned seventy, we students threw a surprise party to honor her. At the next yoga class she stood at the front of the room and announced, "I'm old." We all sat listening quietly in *Sukhasana* (Seated Cross-Legged Pose). Then she pointed out one of the students, a fellow teacher, and said, "And you're old, too," which led to much laughter. She went on to say that she is not *getting* old, she *is* old and that it is okay. As someone capable of leading advanced classes and much revered by her many students, she certainly made being old look more than okay.

I've always been drawn to older people, whether the difference in age was five or thirty years. I realized they had experiences that interested me. Much of my personal growth came through a natural apprenticeship system, thanks to the generosity of my more senior companions. They were willing to share afternoon tea and go for long, contemplative walks where wisdom was openly and freely passed along. So it feels like the perfection of nature's cycle when I am now able to give back to senior adults as a yoga instructor and massage therapist.

Many of my senior yoga students are alone and independent, and it is these students who are often most willing to take on new challenges. "Reach up into *Urdhva Hastasana* (a pose in which the arms are stretched high above the head) as if you're going for the highest shelf in your kitchen," I tell them. If they can't reach it for themselves, who else is going to bring down that vase?

When I moved to rural central Vermont in 2003, I applied for a grant to cover the start-up costs for a seniors yoga class. My application was accepted, and this led to my creating a study on the benefits of yoga for seniors. I established baseline measurements and demonstrated the benefits of a yoga practice for older adults by collecting before and after data from a twelve-week program.

An eclectic group of retired farm wives and others had responded to a survey intended to gauge interest in a seniors yoga class. At first their attention span was scattered, but over the twelve-week period the classes continued, and gradually the focus that came to this group was striking. These new-to-yoga students, in their eighties and early nineties, could practice asana and *pranayama* undisturbed by the comings and goings of other people using the shared facility where the classes were held. Although benefits in function, flexibility, and strength were easily documented, this mental shift—so observable, so important—could not be.

Patanjali's *Yoga Sutras* emphasize this mental shift in the first chapter, Sutra I.II: *"Yogah cittavrtti nirodhah."* ("Yoga is the cessation of the fluctuations of consciousness.") With the practice of yoga, this peace of mind can still be found later in life, even after the loss of a spouse, changes in health, and other landmark events have occurred.

> *Through the practice of yoga we intentionally*
> *create an impression or imprint upon ourselves, mind,*
> *body and soul, that can effect our samskaras*
> *[impressions left by past or current habits that influence*
> *our behavior] and can profoundly influence*
> *the direction of our lives.*
>
> **Leigh Milne**

I find much joy in teaching yoga to senior adults. As individuals they bring incredible life stories to the classroom. Often before beginning our class with a ten-minute *prana* (breathing) exercise, students will engage in a short exchange of public announcements and discussion about the health and well-being of loved ones. Newspaper clippings are brought in, jokes shared, readings offered. Once I begin instruction, attention is given fully to the yoga practice. *Tapas* (conscious effort) pervades for the next hour.

Much significant information was gleaned from the study data collected. Yoga has been found to benefit older adults with increases in balance averaging 75 percent over a twelve-week period. A senior student says she can climb stairs better than she used to, and I can reply, "Well, you've had an increase in quadriceps strength of 50 percent and in hamstring strength of 44 percent as a result of your twice-weekly yoga classes."

Ellen, a seventy-five-year-old woman with Parkinson's disease, has become an accomplished student. Ellen was featured in a newsletter about

Parkinson's when she showed her neurologist a photograph of herself hanging in Rope *Sirsasana* (Headstand). I took that photo after Ellen had been practicing yoga for one year.

Therapeutic Laughter

Many yoga classes are offered exclusively for seniors. This is because the seniors have a better sense of humor and more tolerance than the younger folks. The seniors were always joking and willing to try anything once, so it became necessary to separate them and make a class where they could "let loose." Humor is necessary for life and for yoga, too.

As we age, loss of muscle mass and strength is a common occurrence, partially due to hormonal changes and largely to do with disuse. Muscles must be used to stay strong, and the first to go are the major muscles of ambulation. These are the quadriceps, which lift your thighs for walking and climbing stairs, and the triceps on the back upper arms, which are needed to push up from sitting or lying. Weak back muscles and short chest muscles lead to poor posture—and not just for seniors.

A modified yoga sequence will build strength, improve posture, and make everything else more fun because of it. Yoga is most beneficial when studied in earnest with an experienced teacher.

Leigh Milne, yoga teacher who
specializes in teaching seniors

SAM DWORKIS

The Catch-22 of Younger Yoga Teachers

*S*am Dworkis has been a student and teacher of yoga for over thirty years. He is the author of ExTension and Recovery Yoga: Yoga for Injured, Chronically Ill, and Aging Students. *His website Extensionyoga.com, is a wealth of information on teaching yoga to older students and those with a chronic illness. You would not know it from being in his classes, but Sam himself is in recovery from a serious illness. The following is excerpted from his article entitled "The Paradox of the Younger Yoga Teacher," available at www.extensionyoga.com.*

I recently began teaching a new student who is spending her winters in Florida. At age sixty-one, she's been taking yoga classes with various younger teachers. Although she is in extremely good shape and a willing student, much to her dismay she hasn't yet found a yoga teacher with whom she feels comfortable. Although she can basically do what's asked of her, she's always felt as if she were being pushed too hard. Probably because she is in such good shape, all her younger teachers have been encouraging her to "try harder" and to stretch deeper.

Don't get me wrong. Younger yoga teachers are wonderful. They have the energy and exuberance of youth, and they teach yoga because they want to do something positive to help other people. That being said, many younger yoga teachers "teach from their own perspective," rather than from the perspective of their students. Although teachers might "adapt" yoga exercises for their older and chronically ill and injured students, they still often encourage them to go too far. Taken to the opposite extreme, out of caution many teachers will not encourage them to go far enough.

And herein is the Catch-22 of younger yoga teachers: Because they are young, because they are dedicated and energetic, because they have such a strong desire to help, and because of their own direct experience that comes from their own vigorous yoga practice, they will often push their older or their chronically ill or injured students too far. On the other hand, there are legions of younger teachers who, out of caution or from the lack of education, experience, or confidence, will limit the progress of their students by discouraging them from going far enough.

In both cases, older or chronically ill or injured students lose. To be fair however, students who are advised against going far enough can, in many ways, still reap benefits through yoga, although they will still come short of being able to "maximize their potential."

Younger yoga teachers can help all of their students by studying anatomy, physiology, and kinesiology; by learning the nature of soft tissue and how and why it changes as people age, or become chronically ill or injured; and by taking seminars designed to increase their knowledge of how to work with chronically ill, injured, or aging students.

Education is only half the picture. The other half is for younger yoga teachers to develop an experiential feeling through their own practice, of practicing yoga the way they think their older and chronically ill and injured students should practice, by experimenting within their own practice . . . learning how to "get more by doing less." Although it is easier said than done, learning how to practice as their students practice can help a younger yoga instructor to become a much better teacher.

CHAPTER 11

Yoga Sequences for Healthy Aging

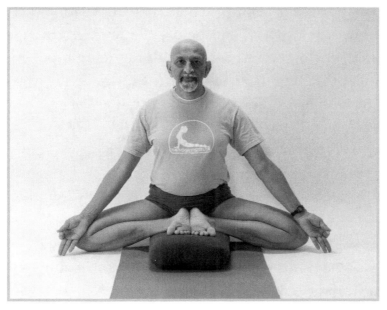

Ramanand Patel demonstrates an advanced variation of Bound-Angle Pose.

*I practice for the joy of setting aside
the practical demands of life and learning
more about peace and the art of being.*

Mary Dunn, senior teacher at the
Iyengar Institute of New York, *Fit Yoga*

This chapter presents a series of basic yoga poses for healthy aging. As we grow older, the order, or *sequence*, in which poses are practiced, becomes increasingly important. Yoga poses are practiced in relationship to each other, in a way that considers the anatomical and physiological effect of the previous pose and prepares the body for the next pose. For example, before turning your body completely upside down (head below the level of the heart and feet up in the air) you prepare by practicing a pose such as Downward-Facing Dog Pose or a Standing Forward Bend Pose, in which the head is below the level of the heart, but the feet are still on the ground. The older we are, the more we need to warm up and practice easier poses before those that are more challenging.

Many yoga poses can be practiced safely on their own. These include restful, restorative poses such as Legs Up the Wall Pose, basic seated poses such as Bound-Angle Pose, and lying-down leg stretches in which you are stretching your legs with a strap or holding your big toe.

When practicing a sequence of poses to help prevent or cope with a health problem, keep in mind that every yoga pose has a multitude of effects on all systems of the body. The experiences of longtime yoga practitioners show that certain poses and sequences of poses act as a tonic for the healthy functioning of certain body systems or organs. Equally important is the overall positive and holistic effect of yoga on the mind, body, and spirit.

Note: *The poses described in this chapter are basic poses that most older beginners can practice safely on their own. The more advanced postures demonstrated in this book are best learned under the guidance of a yoga teacher who can provide specific, individualized instructions and adjustments. Appendix D lists books that give more detailed instructions. Iyengar's book* Yoga: The Path to Holistic Health *illustrates sequences of poses to treat or prevent over eighty ailments.*

Practice in bare feet on a nonslippery surface. Take your time. It is better to do a few poses well than to rush through too many. In all poses—and in your daily life—keep your breath flowing, your jaw and face relaxed, abdomen soft, chest open, and spine elongated.

I expect my practice to continue to be
an ever-expanding source of wonder, delight
and magical power for me for many years to come.
I don't foresee physical limitations of old age impeding
my spiritual unfoldment in the least. In fact, I feel
that as I get older, the depth of my practice will become
more and more profoundly rich. With every passing
month, my yoga practice just gets better!

John Friend, founder of
Anusara Yoga, *Fit Yoga*

Three Essential Poses

- **Stand** every day in bare feet with the back of your body against a wall. The wall helps everyone, especially older beginners, to stand as firm and erect as a mountain with both feet firmly planted on the earth. Most people find it easier to balance their body weight equally between both legs if the feet are slightly apart. Keep your legs straight, feet parallel, and stretch your shoulders back and down the wall. Become aware of your breath, and allow your body and mind to come completely into the present moment. In yoga this is known as Mountain Pose, *Tadasana*. Mountain Pose is the foundation of all the standing poses. It can also be practiced with the arms stretching upward.

- **Sit** on the floor every day, with the back of your body against a wall or chair. The legs can be loosely crossed (Easy or Cross-Legged Pose, *Sukhasana*), or the soles of the feet can be together (Bound-Angle Pose, *Baddha Konasana*), or you can practice sitting with the feet wide apart. This helps ensure that you do not lose the ability to sit comfortably on the floor.

- **Lie** on the floor every day for at least ten minutes in Deep Relaxation Pose, also called Corpse Pose, *Savasana*. This will relieve stress and passively stretch the chest muscles and help correct a rounded upper back. Be sure to place a folded blanket under the head and a firmly rolled towel under the neck if you have a rounded back. (See Chapter 12 for further information on this important pose.)

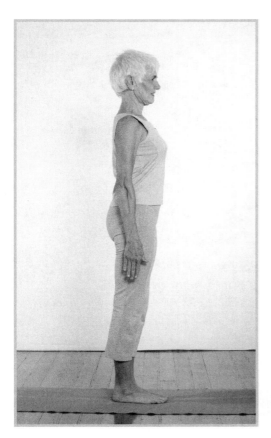

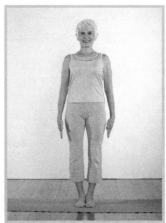

Stand with the weight of your body distributed evenly between the front of your feet and your heels. Practicing near a wall will help you to correct postural problems and stand steady in daily life.

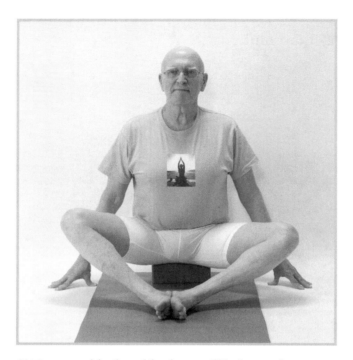

Sitting on a block or blankets will help you keep your back straight and sit comfortably in Bound-Angle Pose.

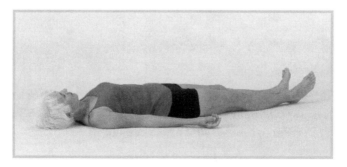

Deep Relaxtion Pose

Your Daily Yoga Vitamin

Most students find it helpful to have at least one short, well-rounded sequence they can practice safely at home. I refer to the following sequence of four poses as "The Daily Yoga Vitamin," your MDR (minimum daily requirement) of yoga.

The following sequence will help ensure that you have the minimum strength needed in your legs and arms to maintain independence. This sequence builds strength and improves your posture and breathing, all of which make daily life more enjoyable.

- Downward-Facing Dog Pose with a Chair
- Upward-Facing Dog Pose with a Chair
- Chair Pose at the Wall
- Wide-Angle Standing Forward Bend Pose

Downward-Facing Dog Pose with a Chair (Adho Mukha Svanasana)

- Put a sturdy, level chair against a wall. Stand with your feet hip width apart. Bend forward and position your hands on the front edge of the chair seat. Keeping your hands on the chair, step back about three feet until your arms are straight. Press your thigh bones and bottom back until you feel a good stretch.

- Breathe calmly and freely. Smile so that your face muscles relax. Stay in the pose for about one minute.

- To come out, step your feet toward the chair, inhale as

INSTRUCTIONS

you bend your knees and stand up. Sit down in the chair for a few moments if you need to rest.

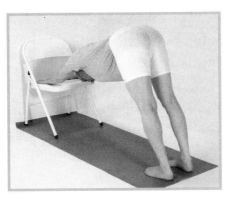

Downward-Facing Dog Pose, with a Chair

This pose strengthens the triceps and quadriceps and gives a rejuvenating stretch to the spine and back of the legs. Tall people and those who are very stiff can experiment with placing the hands on a higher surface.

Upward-Facing Dog Pose with a Chair (Urdhva Mukha Svanasana)

- Begin in Downward-Facing Dog Pose with hands on the chair seat. To move into Upward-Facing Dog Pose, change the positioning of your hands so that they firmly grip the seat sides.

- On an inhalation, come onto the balls of your feet and keep your arms straight as you bring your hips and pubic bone toward the chair. Lift your head upward so that you are looking forward, being careful to keep your neck relaxed. Lift your chest and roll your shoulders back and down. Keep the arms and legs strong and straight. Now exhale, lift your bottom toward the ceiling and stretch back into Downward-Facing Dog Pose.

Tip: *Put a folded sticky mat over the seat to lightly pad the heels of your hands. Repetitions of the Downward- and Upward-Facing Dog sequence will build strength in your wrists, arms, and shoulders and will gently familiarize your wrists with weight bearing so that you can safely practice these poses from the floor.*

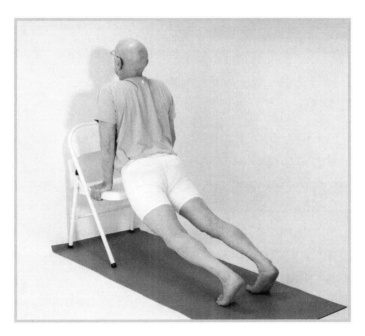

Upward-Facing Dog Pose, **Urdhva Mukha Svanasana,** *with a Chair.*

Chair Pose at the Wall (**Utkatasana**)

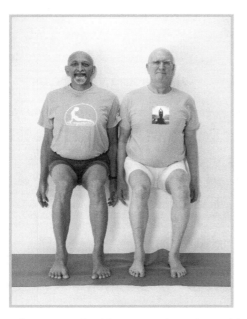

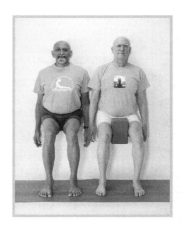

Pressing the inner thighs against a block helps keep the feet, knees, and thigh bones in alignment.

Chair Pose builds strength in the ankles and thighs and helps keep the knees healthy.

• Stand in Mountain Pose with your back against a wall, feet facing straight ahead, hip width apart. Keep your back pressing against the wall as you bend your knees and step about one and a half feet away from the wall (more if you have long legs). Slide your back down the wall until your thighbones are parallel (or almost parallel) to the floor. Your knees should be directly above your heels. If your knees are beyond your heels, move your feet farther from the wall. Press your back firmly into the wall for support so that your chest is open, shoulders back and down. (Viewed from the side the pose looks like you are sitting on an invisible chair.)

• Your hands can be by your side, as illustrated, or on your thighs. As your strength improves, practice the pose with the arms stretching up, palms facing each other.

Tip: *In my classes for seniors, we practice this pose between a pair of wall ropes. Older beginners with tight shoulders find it difficult to keep their elbows straight. Holding onto the upper ropes as you bend your knees gives a beautiful stretch to the spine, shoulders, and arms while at the same time strengthening the quadriceps and triceps and improving posture.*

Caution: *Students with knee problems should bend the knees only so far as there is no pain. Build up time in the pose gradually from half a minute to two minutes. Repeat rather than strain. Breathe peacefully, smile, and keep the throat and face relaxed as you welcome the feeling of the quadriceps strengthening!*

One More Caution: *If you have high blood pressure or heart problems, do not raise your arms above your head in Chair Pose or other standing poses.*

Wide-Angle Standing Forward Bend Pose
(Prasarita Padotanasana)

• Place a chair with a folded blanket or bolster or other support about two feet in front of you. Step your feet three to four feet apart, heels a little wider apart than your toes. Keeping your legs straight by lifting up your front thigh muscles (quadriceps), bend slowly forward from your hip hinge. Depending on your leg flexibility,

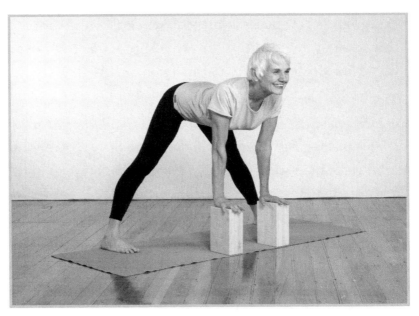

Placing your hands on a chair or blocks and looking up, will help you lengthen you spine in Wide-Angle Standing Forward Bend **Prasarita Padotanasana.**

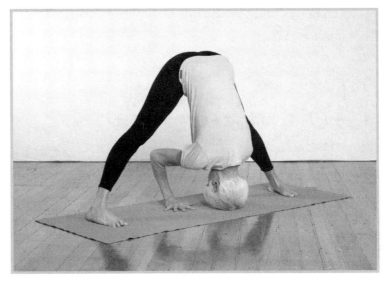

Place a chair or other support under your head if it does not touch the floor.

place your fingertips or palms on a chair, two blocks or other height, arms straight as illustrated, head looking up toward the ceiling. This action both stabilizes your knee joints and allows the hamstring muscles at the back of the thighs to release.

• After lengthening your spine, as illustrated, gently relax the head down. Resting your head on a chair or block brings your head below the level of your heart and has a soothing effect on your brain and nervous system. Stay in the pose about half a minute, increasing the time gradually.

To come up, place your hands on your legs, and inhale deeply as you return to standing upright. Feel the calming, soothing effect of this pose.

Benefits: *Standing Forward Bends stretch the back of the body. They are restful for the heart and increase circulation to the head. Practiced with the spine concave, they help strengthen the pelvic floor and prevent urinary incontinence.*

This well-rounded sequence, if practiced daily, will strengthen and stretch the muscles you need for activities of daily living.

The Master Pose for Reversing the Aging Process: Downward-Facing Dog

After you become familiar with Downward-Facing Dog Pose with a chair, you can practice the pose with your hands on the floor. Downward-Facing Dog Pose is named for the way dogs and other animals naturally stretch their bodies several times a day. It can be practiced by itself, or before, or after, any of the individual poses or sequences of poses described in this chapter. Downward-Facing Dog Pose is a halfway inverted position that almost everyone can safely practice. Even octogenarians who may not have stretched for many years can begin to enjoy this pose very early in their practice. This pose inverts the internal organs and increases blood flow to the head. A weight-bearing pose, it strengthens the hands, wrists, arms, and shoulders. Downward- and Upward-Facing Dog poses work together to remove stiffness from the shoulder joints, wrists, hands, and fingers. The whole spinal column is lengthened, abdominal muscles are strengthened, and neck tension is released.

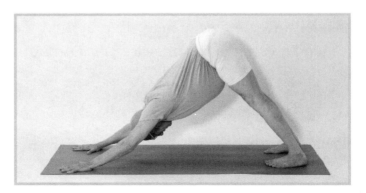

Give your body a rejuvenating stretch in Downward-Facing Dog Pose every day!

INSTRUCTIONS

Downward-Facing Dog Pose

- Begin on your hands and knees, on a non-slippery surface. Position your knees slightly behind your hips, toes curled under, your feet and knees hip width apart. Place your hands slightly in front of your shoulders, shoulder distance apart. Spread all ten fingers wide apart and press both hands down into the floor.

- On an exhalation, lift your buttocks toward the ceiling, partially straightening your legs, so that your body forms a high upside down V or pyramid shape. Press your hands deeper into the floor, stretching the thigh bones back. After stretching for a few breaths with your heels lifted, press your heels down toward the floor. Breathe smoothly, naturally. Release, come back to kneeling on all fours. Lower your bottom back toward your heels and rest in Child's Pose.

Caution: *Do not practice with your hands on the floor if you have glaucoma or retinal problems or if you suffer from a hiatal hernia. Do not stay in the pose if your back hurts or if you feel unusual pressure in the head or dizziness.*

About Wrist Strain: *If your wrists are painful, place a folded sticky mat or yoga wedge underneath the heel of your hands, so the wrist is slightly elevated and supported by the extra cushioning. (Also see the information about Gripitz, pages 51–52.) If you have serious wrist problems—like carpal tunnel syndrome or previous fracture or surgery sites that are stiff and painful—please consult your healthcare provider before attempting weight-bearing poses. (Also see page 250, Downward-Facing Dog Pose with a Chair.)*

Standing poses safely strengthen the skeletal system and remove joint and muscle stiffness. The back, hips, knees, neck, and shoulders all gain strength and mobility with regular practice. They also improve circulation and breathing, stimulate digestion, regulate the kidneys, and relieve constipation. Oxygen is drawn into the body, removing lethargy and fatigue. The breath flows freely, and the whole body becomes energized.

Standing poses, practiced with the back of the body supported by the horse, wall, or other support, conserve energy, improve body alignment, and increase the benefits. Depending on your height, about six feet of empty wall space is ideal. If wall space is not available, use a windowsill or kitchen counter. Standing poses can also be practiced facing the wall.

A Sequence of
Four Standing Poses

- Extended Triangle Pose *(Utthita Trikonasana)* at the Wall

- Warrior II Pose *(Virabhadrasana II)* at the Wall

- Extended Side-Angle Pose *(Utthita Parsvakonasana)* at the Wall

- Half-Moon Pose *(Ardha Chandrasana)* at the Wall

Extended Triangle Pose
(Utthita Trikonasana) *at the Wall*

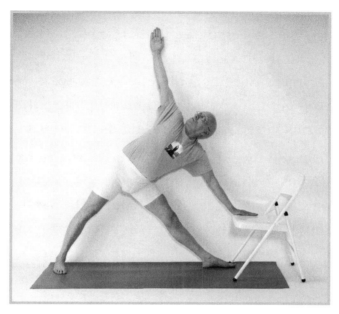

Practicing Supported Extended Triangle Pose with the wall and a chair helps assure that you move from the hip joint and extend your torso evenly.

- Stand tall with your posture open, shoulders relaxed, near a wall or other support. Step your feet about four feet apart (depending on your flexibility and the length of your legs), keeping your feet facing forward and your heels close to the wall.

- Anchor your feet to the earth by pressing the soles of your feet deep into the floor. Keep your legs straight by lifting up your thigh muscles. Allow your body to become taller and taller, lengthening your spine upward.

INSTRUCTIONS

- Raise your arms to shoulder level, palms facing down, and stretch your arms out from the center of your body in opposite directions. Breathe softly and smoothly.

- When you feel centered in this position, turn the left foot slightly inward and the right foot out 90 degrees. Line up the right heel directly in line with the center of the left arch. If you find it difficult to turn the feet with the arms raised, place your hands on your hips.

- Inhale, and on exhalation stretch to the right from the hip joint, so that your torso stretches sideways as a unit toward your right leg. Place your right hand on a chair, as illustrated, to help lengthen your spine and avoid straining your knees. Make sure your right kneecap is turning toward your right little toe.

- Extend your left arm up, in line with your right arm, palm facing forward. If you feel unusual strain in your shoulder, try placing your left hand on your hip or hold onto a wall rope or other support.

- Stay in the pose for several breaths, keeping your legs straight, your shoulders stretching down the back and your neck relaxed. Come out of the pose on an inhalation, keeping your body close to the wall. Turn your feet to face forward. Relax back into the wall, and pause for a moment to feel the effects of the pose.

- Repeat on the other side.

- Step your feet back together, and stand tall against the wall.

Warrior II Pose
(Virabhadrasana II) *at the Wall or Other Support*

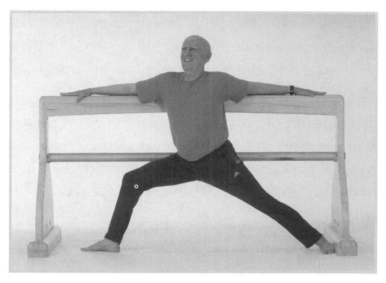

Practicing Warrior II Pose, **Virabhadrasana II,** *with the support of the horse or a wall will help you keep your upper body centered.*

• Stand with your back against a wall and use the wall to help you maintain your awareness of good posture, just as in Triangle Pose.

• Separate your feet approximately four- to four-and-a-half feet apart, with feet parallel. Stretch your arms out in line with your shoulders, palms down, fingers straight. Turn your left foot slightly inward and your right foot out 90 degrees. Keep your right heel in line with the arch of your left foot.

• Exhale, and bend your right knee so that your leg forms a right angle. Stretch your arms in both directions, stretch your shoulders back and down, in contact with the wall or other support, to open your chest. Keep your abdomen lifted but soft, and gaze at your right hand. Keep your back leg straight and press both feet strongly into the floor. Hold the pose long enough so that you feel your legs strengthening, but not so long that you collapse! Keep your breath flowing freely, lips closed softly.

• To come out of the pose, straighten your right leg as you come up and turn your feet so they are back to the original parallel position. Turn your right foot in slightly and your left foot out 90 degrees. Repeat on the left side.

Benefits: *Warrior II Pose strengthens the back and legs, develops strength and stamina, and gives an intense stretch to the groin.*

Note: *In the beginning, you may not be ready to take such a wide stance or to bend the knee to a right angle. Practice with a shorter stride until the inner thighs lengthen and the hips open. Check that your stance is wide enough so that your bent knee does not move past your heel.*

Extended Side-Angle Pose
(Utthita Parsvakonasana) *at the Wall*

• Stand with your back against a wall and use the wall to help you maintain your awareness of good posture, just as in Triangle Pose. Keep your arms, shoulder blades, and buttocks in contact with the wall. Place a block within reach to the right of your mat.

• Separate your feet about four feet apart, feet facing parallel. Stretch your arms out in line with your shoulders, palms down, fingers straight. Turn your left foot slightly inward and your right foot out 90 degrees. Keep your right heel in line with the arch of your left foot. Keep your legs straight, kneecaps lifted, and both feet firmly anchored to the earth.

• Stretch your arms in both directions. Stretch your shoulders back and down, holding onto the support of the trestle (horse) or a counter or windowsill. Exhale and bend the right leg into a right angle, keeping your upper body in the center as much as possible and strongly anchoring through your back leg. Move into Extended Side-Angle Pose, lowering your fingertips to the floor or block. Beginners can place a block in front or back of the foot.

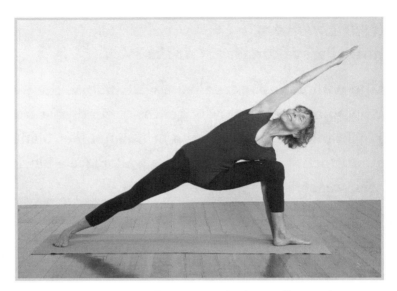

Practicing Extended Side-Angle Pose with the wall or other support will help prepare you to practice the pose with good alignment in the center of the room.

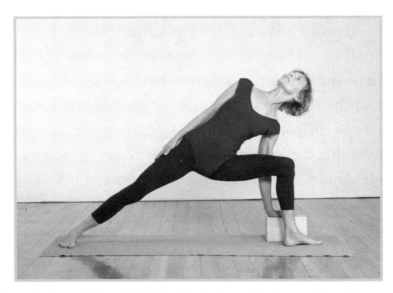

In this variation of Extended Side-Angle Pose the bottom hand is on a block and the top hand is on the back thigh to help keep the body in alignment.

Half-Moon Pose (**Ardha Chandrasana**) *at the Wall*

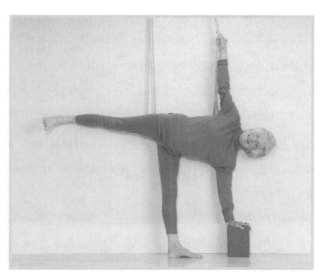

Use a wall or other support to help you balance in Half-Moon Pose. Stretch in all directions so that the pose sparkles!

• Standing against the wall or other support, separate your feet four to four-and-a-half feet apart as in Extended Triangle Pose. Stretch your arms out in line with your shoulders. Turn your left foot slightly inward and right foot out 90 degrees, and, keeping the back of your head and both shoulders on the wall, come into Extended Triangle Pose. Bend your right knee and place the fingertips of your right hand on a chair seat or block, a foot or more in front of your right foot.

• Exhale, and shift your weight forward and onto your right foot. Lift your left leg as your right leg straightens. Stay close to the wall so that when you move into the pose the back of your head, both shoulders, your whole back, your left and right buttocks, your lifted leg, and the heel of your lifted foot all press back against the wall.

• Keep both legs straight. Lift your left arm toward the ceiling, palm facing forward. Keep your abdomen soft, with your pelvis and chest turning toward the ceiling.

• Exhale back to Triangle Pose and inhale up. Turn your right foot in and your left foot out and repeat on the opposite side.

Benefits: *Half-Moon Pose increases circulation and massages the organs of the abdomen and pelvis. It is a key pose for lengthening the spine, strengthening your back, and opening and strengthening the hips, legs, ankles, and feet.*

A Sequence of Two Seated Poses

• Bound-Angle Pose *(Baddha Konasana)*
• Seated Wide-Angle Pose *(Upavistha Konasana)*

A lifetime of sitting in chairs causes stiffness in the hips and knees. Most people unaccustomed to sitting on the floor tend to slump backward and collapse their chests. By sitting on two firmly folded blankets, a block, or a bolster, students learn what it feels like to sit with the chest open. The stiffer you are in the hips, the thicker the height under your bottom should be. If you feel strain in your knees, try placing a folded blanket or other support under your knees.

INSTRUCTIONS

Bound-Angle Pose—Cobbler's Pose (Baddha Konasana)

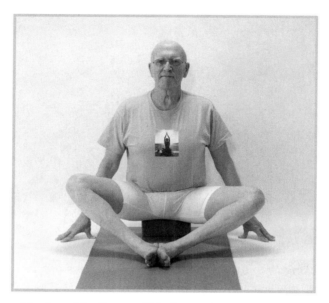

Sitting on a block or blankets will help you keep your back straight and sit comfortably in Bound-Angle Pose.

- Sit on one or two folded blankets, a bolster, or a yoga block. Bend your knees and bring your feet toward your pubic bone. Join the soles of your feet together. Place your fingertips behind your hips, lengthen your spine up toward the ceiling, lift and open your chest, and press your legs toward the floor.

- Keeping the lift in your spine, clasp your fingers around your feet. Keep your abdomen soft, face relaxed, breath flowing, and allow your pelvis to open and your groin muscles to relax. Stay in the pose for a few minutes, gradually increasing the length of time.

Seated Wide-Angle Pose (**Upavistha Konasana**)

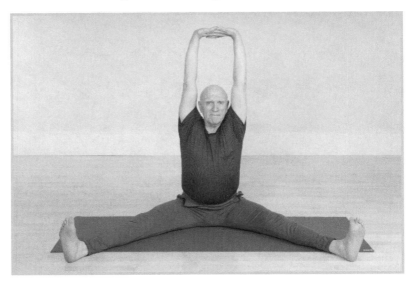

Interlocking the fingers and stretching the arms upward helps lengthen the spine and open the shoulders in Seated Wide-Angle Pose.

- Sit on the floor, on a folded blanket if necessary, to align the spine and pelvis.

- Separate your legs as wide apart as you can without causing discomfort. Keep your heels in line with each other.

- Place the fingertips on the floor behind the hips, and stretch your spine up. You can also stretch your arms up, as illustrated

- Stay on the center of your heels, and press the backs of your legs into the floor. Make sure your knee caps are facing up.

• Relax your abdomen. Focus on opening and widening the pelvis.

Benefits: *Seated poses help keep the knee and hip joints healthy. The regular practice of Bound-Angle Pose increases the flow of blood to the abdomen, pelvis, and back. It helps to treat urinary tract disorders and to keep the kidneys and prostate gland healthy. You can practice sitting upright in Seated Wide-Angle Pose and Seated Bound-Angle Pose at anytime, even after eating. I highly recommend sitting in these two poses every day for at least five minutes.*

A Sequence of Two Lying-Down Poses

• Lying-Down Big-Toe Pose I and II (Supta Padangusthasana I and II)
• Lying-Down Twist or Twist-Around-the-Belly Pose (Jathara Parivartanasana)

Lying-Down Big-Toe Pose I and II (Supta Padangusthasana I and II)

• Before lying down, loop a long, adjustable yoga strap around your back.

• Lie on your back and slip the right leg through the strap. Straighten your leg up toward the ceiling.

• Adjust the length of the strap so that you feel the back of the leg stretching.

Lying-Down Big-Toe Pose I and II
(Supta Padangusthasana I and II)

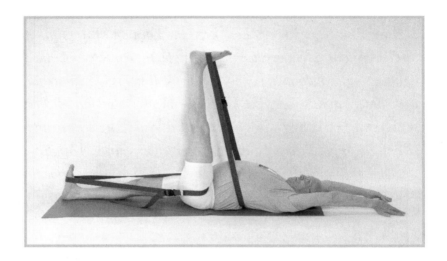

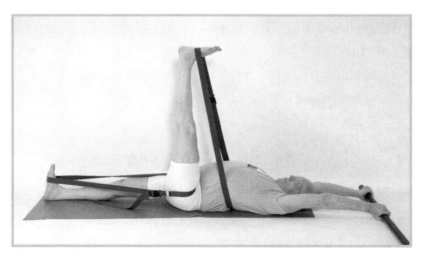

Lying-Down Big-Toe Pose I. Stretching with two long straps creates traction and helps ease back pain. Place the second strap around top of thigh and ball of the opposite foot.

The photos shown here illustrate how to use yoga straps and other props to keep your whole body in alignment when practicing Lying-Down Big-Toe Pose and variations of it.

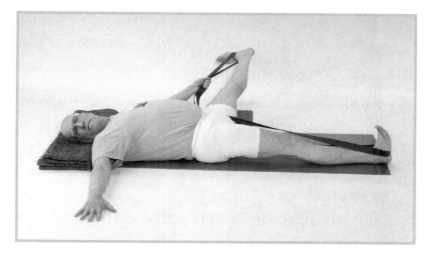

Lying-Down Big-Toe Pose II, leg to the side.

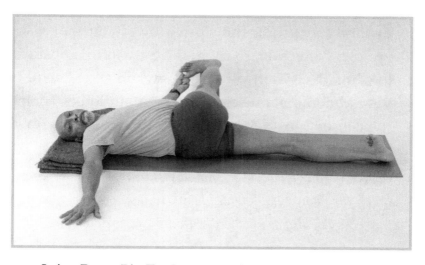

Lying-Down Big-Toe Pose, Revolved or Twist variation.

• Keep your hips level (both buttock bones on the floor) as you slowly stretch your leg out to the side, as illustrated (Lying-Down Big-Toe Pose II).

Benefits: *Removes stiffness in the legs and hips.*

Lying-Down Twist or Twist-Around-the-Belly Pose (Jathara Parivartanasana)

• Lie on your back on the floor with your knees bent, feet flat on the floor, your upper body and lower body in line. Place a folded blanket under your head if needed to keep the forehead and chin level so that your head does not tilt back. Bring your arms in line with your shoulders, palms up, hands actively stretching away from each other to open your chest.

• Lift your hips off the floor to move them gently to the left. Lower your hips back to the floor. Bend your knees toward your chest, and slowly lower your knees in the opposite direction, to the right. Stay in this posture for a few breaths. When you feel ready, on an exhalation use your abdominal muscles to bring your knees back to the center. Move your hips to the right before slowly lowering your knees to the left.

Note: *If you feel back or shoulder strain, or if your knees do not touch the floor, place a folded blanket under your legs, as illustrated. The pose can also be practiced with the arm stretching over your head.*

Benefits: *Gentle floor twists help prevent and relieve lower back pain caused by muscle tension. They help relieve indigestion and*

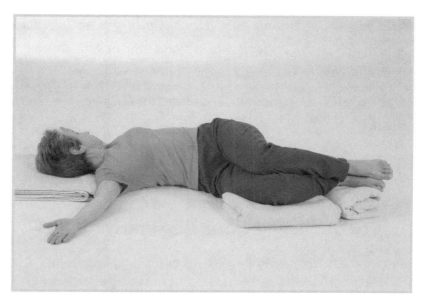

Lying-Down Twist or Twist-Around-the-Belly Pose (**Jathara Parivartanasana**), *with both knees bent.*

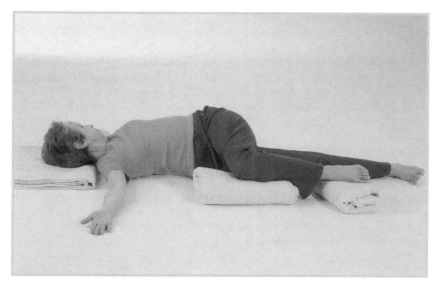

Variation of Lying-Down Bent-Knee Twist, with one leg straight.

help tone the abdominal area. The abdomen gets an internal massage in this pose. Gentle floor twists ease tension and stiffness in the neck and shoulders.

Caution: *Check with your healthcare professional before practicing this pose if you have disk disease in your lower back.*

A Sequence of Four Restorative Poses

- Supported Bridge Pose *(Setu Bandha Sarvangasana)*
- Legs Up the Wall Pose *(Viparita Karani)*
- Supported Legs Up the Wall Pose *(Viparita Karani)*
- Supported Lying-Down Bound-Angle Pose *(Supta Baddha Konasana)*

Restorative yoga poses are restful, passive poses in which the body is lying still, supported with props. Restorative poses give us the opportunity to be quiet, silent, and in this state of stillness to restore ourselves—physically, mentally, and spiritually. In the restorative poses, the idea is a long stay in the pose, which allows the mind and body to access deeper levels of relaxation and experience what can best be described as divine rest.

It is now well established that prolonged stress accelerates the aging process. Restorative yoga poses trigger a set of physiological changes that allows your body to recover from the effects of stress. Practicing with props is unique in that it is the only form that allows both action and relaxation simultaneously. Action and relaxation are vital for healthy aging because they replenish our energy reserves and rejuvenate the entire body without increasing fatigue.

While getting enough sleep is vital for good health, the normal sleep state does not trigger all the conditions needed for deep relaxation. During sleep we tense our muscles, we dream, and our minds are active. I highly recommend taking a "yoga nap" every day. If you are tired, you may fall asleep and experience a level of rest that is more refreshing than napping in bed or on the couch.

All stress reduction techniques begin with observing the breath. Spend some time practicing slow, deep inhalations and slow, deep exhalations, without straining. Gently quiet the flow of your breath.

Supported Bridge Pose (**Setu Bandha Sarvangasana**)

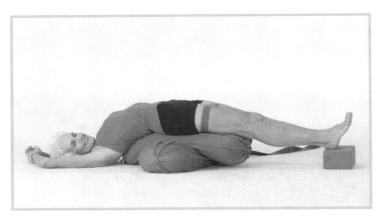

You can't help but smile after practicing Supported Bridge Pose! Adjust the height of your support until your body feels sublimely comfortable.

The photo of Supported Bridge Pose shows one of several ways to place folded blankets or bolsters under the back and legs. The height of the support depends on the length of your torso and the flexibility of your back. (See page 186 for gentle variation of this pose.)

• Sit on the bolsters, either with your legs straight out in front of you or with your feet on the floor on either side of the bolster. Position yourself near one end of the bolster so that when you lie down your head is near the far end. Use the support of your arms as you lie down. Slowly slide off the end until the back of your head and shoulders rest flat on the floor.

• If you had difficulty lowering your shoulders to the floor, either use a lower support or place a folded blanket under your shoulders and head. If your lower back feels strained, try bending your knees and placing your feet on the floor on either side of the bolster. Relax your throat and chin. Lengthen and release your neck.

• When you feel comfortable, close your eyes and cover them with an eye bag. Allow your breath, mind, and heart to slow. Relax your arms out to the side at a comfortable angle, or with your elbows bent and arms relaxing back just above your shoulders.

• Stay in Supported Bridge Pose for five minutes or longer. When you feel ready to come out, remove your eye bag, bend your knees, and slowly turn to your side. Alternatively, you can slide off the bolster in the direction of your head, until your whole back and bottom are on the floor. Relax for a few more breaths with your lower legs supported by the height. Then bend your knees, turn to your side, and sit up slowly.

Benefits: *Supported Bridge Pose is a combination gentle supported backbend and mild inverted position. You can clearly see and feel the opening of the chest and heart area as you place your body in this pose. It is restful for the heart and may help balance blood pressure and hormonal secretions. It has a calming effect on the mind and nervous system and helps prevent and relieve headaches. Placing your head lower than the rest of your body with the chest open is soothing and refreshing and removes lethargy and depression. It also helps drain fluid from the legs after long periods of standing.*

Legs Up the Wall Pose: Yoga's Great Rejuvenator

Legs Up the Wall, practiced with or without support, is a gentle, inverted pose that can be practiced by almost everyone. It is a safe, nonthreatening position that most people can hold long enough so that gravity can return the blood from the extremities to the vital organs.

People who are bedridden can practice this pose by placing a bed against a wall or stacking blankets and pillows on a bed in such a way that the legs can be gently inverted. This pose can help relieve swollen legs and feet.

Supported Legs Up the Wall Pose is known as Yoga's Great Rejuvenator. It is considered the most healing of the yoga restorative poses. When you turn upside down, gravity helps the venous blood—which otherwise tends to pool in the legs—to return easily to the heart. In people whose heart rates are elevated because they have not been receiving an ample supply of blood, this pose reduces the heart rate by improving the blood flow into the chest. In this gentle supported inversion, as in other more active inverted postures, the weight of the blood in the feet, legs, and abdomen stimulates blood pressure receptors in the neck and chest to reduce the constriction of the arteries throughout the body. This reduces blood pressure.

Part of the soothing effect derived from Supported Legs Up the Wall Pose is due to the angle of the torso. Note in the photos how the bolster positioned under the pelvis brings the torso into a gentle supported backbend, while the wall supports the legs. As you lie in the pose, you can imagine that its shape creates an internal waterfall, as the fluid in the legs cascades down to the abdomen and spills over into the chest, toward the heart. This waterfall effect creates a peaceful, soothing sensation.

Practice this daily if your legs and feet swell easily or if you have varicose veins. When you are tired, get in the habit of napping with your legs up the wall to replenish your energy reserves.

An eye bag over the eyes and a sandbag on the feet increase the feeling of relaxation. Note how the position of the bolster causes the rib cage to open and spread. Two firm folded blankets can be used in place of a bolster. The width of the blanket depends somewhat on your height and flexibility. For most people, the edge of the blanket can be placed at the waist. This placement allows the back to curve in such a way that the chest opens and the lower back feels comfortable.

Legs Up the Wall Pose *(Viparita Karani)*

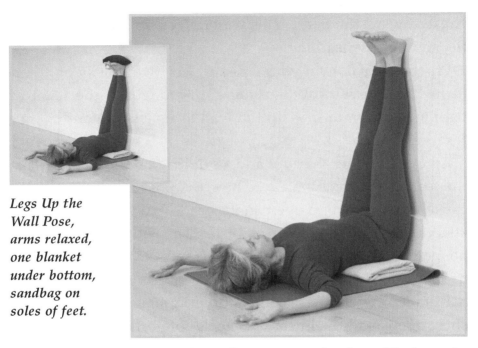

Legs Up the Wall Pose, arms relaxed, one blanket under bottom, sandbag on soles of feet.

Legs Up the Wall Pose, arms relaxed, one blanket under bottom. Gentle variation for beginners.

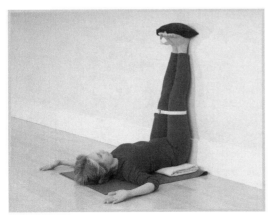

Legs Up the Wall Pose, arms relaxed, one blanket under bottom, sandbag on soles of feet, strap around thighs.

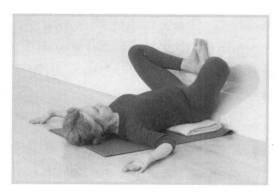

*Legs Up the Wall Pose, arms relaxed, one blanket under bottom, soles of the feet together (Bound Angle Pose, **Baddha Konasana** at the wall).*

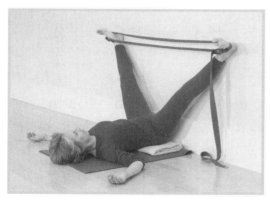

Legs Up the Wall Pose, arms relaxed, one blanket under bottom, feet wide apart. The strap around the feet helps to keep the heels in line but it is perfectly fine to practice this variation of Legs Up the Wall Pose without a strap.

INSTRUCTIONS

If you are unfamiliar with Supported Legs Up the Wall Pose, first try the pose without any support under your bottom. Become familiar with simply relaxing with your legs up on the wall.

If you have difficulty lowering yourself to the floor, you can practice this in bed by positioning one side of your bed right against a bare wall.

• Sit sideways on the floor beside a wall, knees bent, with one shoulder and hip touching the wall. Draw your legs close to your chest. Lower your back to the floor, with your legs bent, keeping your bottom close to the wall. Swing around to bring your legs up the wall, supporting yourself on your elbows and forearms.

• Look at your legs and check that they are in line with your upper body so that you form an L shape. If the backs of your legs are tight, your legs may not touch the wall. If straightening the legs causes you to slide farther away from the wall, try keeping the knees slightly bent. It is more important that your back feels comfortable and that your head is level than that you have your legs right up against the wall.

• If needed, place a folded blanket under your head to keep it level and comfortable. Your neck must feel comfortable, without any tightness or pinching at the nape. If blood flow to the head is obstructed, the brain cannot relax.

• The next step is to practice with one folded blanket within easy reach. Lift your lower back off the floor and place the blanket under your bottom, with your lower back supported.

Note: *Placing folded blankets under your bottom repositions the head so that it rests level on the floor. People with a very rounded upper back (kyphosis) may still need a folded blanket under the head even when the bottom is supported.*

Supported Legs Up the Wall Pose *(Viparita Karani)*

• Place a bolster (or several firm folded blankets) with the long side parallel to the wall, about three to six inches away from the wall. (The distance depends on your height, leg flexibility, and personal preference.)

• Sit sideways on the bolster or blankets with knees bent. Your right hip and side should touch the wall. With the bolster under your bottom, lean back slightly, using the support of your elbows and forearms, and swivel around to take your legs up the wall.

• If leg stiffness prevents you from being close to the wall, pull the bolster toward you so that your lower back, lower ribs, and bottom are comfortably supported by the bolster and your shoulders and head rest comfortably on the floor.

• You should be supported from the back of the pelvis to the lowest ribs; adjust the support if necessary. If you have the sensation that you are falling off the bolster toward your head, scoot your bottom toward the wall, slightly over the bolster and toward the floor. Stretch your shoulders down the back to help open your chest.

• Straighten the legs up the wall. Stretch the inner and outer sides of your legs evenly, and allow the weight of your legs to move down toward your sitting bones. The weight of a sandbag placed across the soles of the feet will help you to accomplish this and makes the posture even more relaxing.

Supported Legs Up the Wall Pose *(Viparita Karani)*

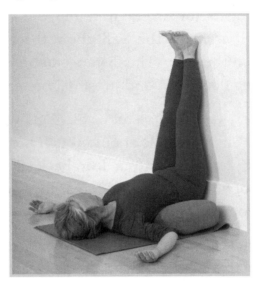

Supported Legs Up the Wall Pose, bolster under bottom, eye bag over eyes, arms overhead.

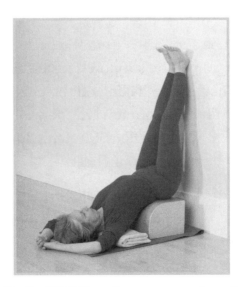

Supported Legs Up the Wall Pose for more experienced students, using a special prop that opens the chest and elevates the body even more.

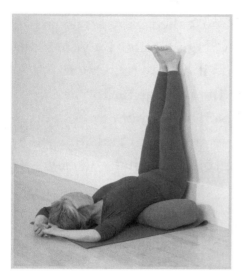

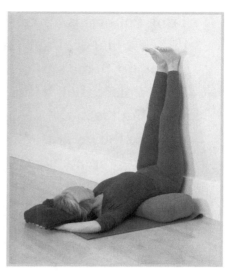

*Variation, arms overhead with
fingers touching.*

*Variation, sandbag over hands.
Weights placed strategically on the
body make all Restorative Poses
even more relaxing.*

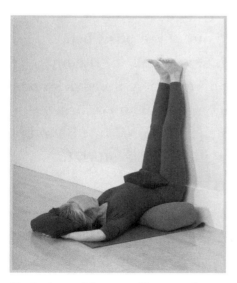

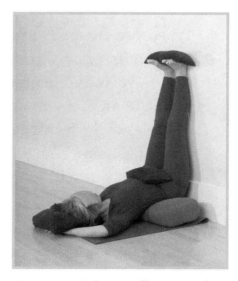

*Variation with a sandbag on the
abdomen.*

*Variation with a sandbag on soles
of the feet.*

INSTRUCTIONS

- Bring your arms into a T shape (called baby arms or cactus arms) or simply allow them to relax by your side, palms up. Some students find it deeply relaxing to lightly place their hands on the rib cage for the first few minutes in the pose, which helps them to feel and observe the breath. Allow the arms and hands to end up in a completely passive position so that you can totally let go.

- When you feel comfortable, close your eyes and cover them with an eye bag. Observe the rise and fall of your breath. Allow your heart and chest area to relax and open. Stay in the pose for ten minutes or longer.

- Follow Supported Legs Up the Wall Pose with a few minutes of gently stretching your legs on the wall, as illustrated on page 281, before you slowly sit up.

- When you are ready to come out of the pose, bend your knees, press your feet into the wall, lift the hips, and move away from the wall until the whole back rests on the floor. Cross your legs on the bolster, or bring the soles of the feet together as in Lying-Down Bound-Angle Pose, and rest. When you feel ready, turn to your right side and sit up.

Note: *If you are tired, it is natural to fall asleep in this pose. If you cannot get comfortable in this pose, try a lower height. Many people with tight hamstrings or sensitive backs initially feel more relaxed with just one blanket. This pose can be a lifesaver and is well worth learning under the guidance of a knowledgeable teacher.*

Wall ropes are a tremendous help in practicing this pose. My new students in their seventies or eighties often use the lower wall ropes to lower themselves to the floor and then they practice this pose between the two ropes. They use the ropes to scoot closer to the wall and to position themselves comfortably on a folded blanket or bolster.

More experienced students with access to wall ropes can practice *Viparita Karani* by positioning a bolster on top of a yoga mat between a set of wall ropes. You stand on the bolster, holding the upper ropes, walk up the wall, and then lower yourself gracefully onto the bolster and into the pose. Be sure to have a teacher supervise you the first time you try it.

Caution: *People with heart problems, neck problems, eye pressure, retinal problems, or hiatal hernia should use caution with all inverted poses. However, Supported Legs Up the Wall Pose is recommended for those with mild hypertension because it can help normalize blood pressure. If you experience discomfort with your legs straight up the wall, experiment with helping your body become accustomed to the pose by first lying down with the lower legs resting on the seat of a chair (a backless yoga chair or folding chair or stool works best). See Chapter 9.*

Supported Lying-Down Bound-Angle Pose (Supta Baddha Konasana)

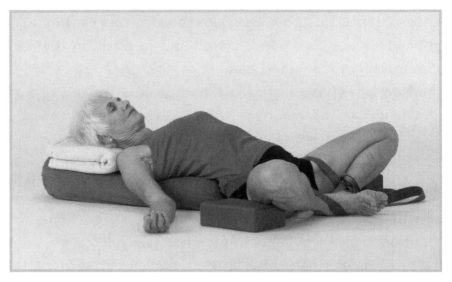

As we grow older, restorative poses like Supported Lying-Down Bound-Angle Pose are increasingly important for reenergizing the body.

- Sit in front of the bolster placed lengthwise behind you, with the soles of your feet together. Have one or two folded blankets at the top of the bolster to create a comfortable support for your head and neck.

- Loop a strap behind your back, at your sacrum (just above your tailbone, not your waist). Bring the strap forward, around your hips, across your shins, and under your feet so that the soles of your feet are secure. Secure the strap in such a way that it is not too tight or too loose. (Ask your teacher to demonstrate this if you have not yet learned it in class.)

- Center your spine on the bolster. Bring the soles of your feet close to your body. Place a folded blanket (or yoga block) under each of your outer thighs. The height of the blankets should adequately support the weight of your legs so that your back and knees relax. Your knees should be level. If one knee is much higher, place extra support under the lower knee. Many people also feel more relaxed with the support of a folded blanket under their forearms. Blankets can be folded lengthwise and carefully positioned to support both the legs and arms.

- Check that the height under your head feels comfortable. Place an eye bag over your eyes. Turn your palms up. Allow your body to soften and relax.

- If you feel discomfort in your back, try repositioning your back on the bolster—you may be too high or too low on the bolster. Use your hands to move the flesh of the buttocks down and away from your waist. If you still feel strain, decrease the height under your back by placing a folded blanket under your bottom.

- When you are comfortable, stay in the pose for ten minutes or longer. Observe the peaceful flow of your breath. To come out of the pose, place your hands under your thighs and bring your legs back together. Remove the strap and straighten your legs, allowing them to fall evenly away from the midline. When you feel ready, bend your knees, turn to your side, and use your hands to help you slowly sit up.

Note: *Some older beginners will prefer to practice this pose with a blanket folded lengthwise to support the length of the spine and head. Others prefer lying flat with the soles of the feet together on top of the bolster.*

Benefits: *Practicing Lying-Down Bound-Angle Pose with support from bolsters and blankets opens the chest, abdomen, and pelvis and allows the body to relax deeply. Extra support under the forearms, knees, and outer thighs makes the pose supremely comfortable and nourishing. This pose is also beneficial to those with high blood pressure, headaches, and breathing problems.*

Additional Inverted Poses for Experienced Students

- Supported Shoulderstand at the Wall
  (*Salamba Sarvangasana*)

- Supported Shoulderstand with a Chair
  (*Salamba Sarvangasana*)

- Supported Half Plow Pose with a Chair
  (*Ardha Halasana*)

Supported Shoulderstand at the Wall (Salamba Sarvangasana)

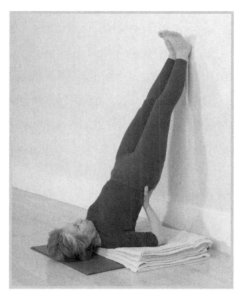

Supported Shoulderstand at the Wall.

The support of a wall or a chair helps you to straighten your back, open your chest, relax, and stay in the pose longer. It is advisable to have a teacher assist you the first few times you practice this.

In Shoulderstand, the back of your head is on the floor, with the shoulders about two to three inches from the edge of the blanket. The purpose of elevating the shoulders on a stack of blankets is to protect the neck. Keep your neck soft and relaxed. In Shoulderstand the cervical vertebrae, the smallest and weakest of the spinal bones, are in a most vulnerable position. The raised platform of folded blankets is used to lift the neck away from the floor.

The bones of the neck should not press into the floor. To avoid injury, do not turn your head in Shoulderstand. Keep your chin in line with your chest.

Prepare a set of three to five folded blankets, with the smooth folded edge toward the center of the room. The blanket should be wide enough to support your shoulders and elbows. Shoulderstand may seem easier without having to prepare by folding all those blankets to support your weight, but the effort is worth it: The weight of the body has a tendency to cause strain and pressure on the neck when you're unaccustomed to it. Your teacher can help you to determine the right number of blankets to use.

- Place the firm, folded blankets near a wall, with the folded edges away from the wall. Have about one to two feet between the wall and the back edge of the blankets. The exact distance away from the wall depends on the length of your torso.

- Sit on the blankets beside a wall, knees bent, with one shoulder and hip touching the wall, as in Legs Up the Wall Pose.

- Shift your weight onto your opposite elbow and shoulder and swivel your trunk around to bring your legs up the wall so that you are lying on your back with your shoulders well supported by the blankets and the back of your neck and head are off the blankets.

- Many beginners inadvertently slip off the blankets when they first try this pose. As in Legs Up the Wall

Pose, you may need to wriggle your bottom closer to the wall so that your shoulders remain on the blankets while your legs are up the wall. If your shoulders fall off the blankets when your bottom is close to the wall, try placing the blankets a little farther away from the wall to accommodate the length of your torso.

• Bend your knees, press the soles of your feet against the wall, and raise your hips and chest off the floor until your back feels straight. Firmly support your back with both hands, bringing your elbows closer together. Make sure your shoulders have remained on the blankets and the back of your head is on the floor. Your neck should feel comfortable without pressure or pain. Do not turn your neck once you are in this position. If you feel comfortable, stay in the pose for a few minutes, gradually increasing your stay. When you are ready to come down, place your hands back on the floor, bend your knees, and gently lower your back and bottom to the floor.

• Relax with your legs up the wall a few more minutes by sliding back off the blankets until your upper back is on the floor. When you feel ready to sit up, bend your knees, turn to your side, and slowly sit up. You also can remain on the floor in a lying position to follow this pose with some gentle floor twists.

Supported Shoulderstand with a Chair
(Salamba Sarvangasana)

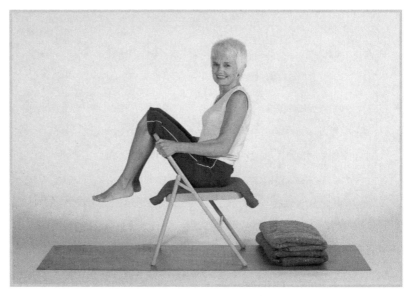

Shoulderstand with chair, sitting on the chair, with legs over the back of the chair.

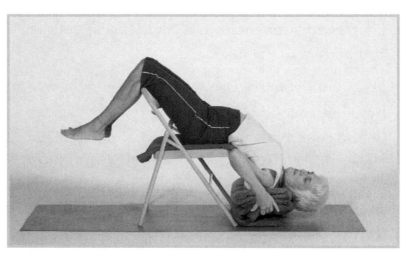

Transition to placing shoulders on folded blanket.

INSTRUCTIONS

- Place a sturdy chair on a nonslippery surface and place a bolster or two folded blankets directly in front of the chair legs to support your shoulders. Place a folded sticky mat or folded blanket over the front edge of the chair seat.

- Sitting on the chair, as illustrated, bring your legs over the back. Holding onto the chair, lower your shoulders to the blankets and the back of your head to the floor.

Benefits: *According to Iyengar, Shoulderstand alleviates hypertension; improves the functioning of the thyroid and parathyroid glands; helps relieve insomnia and soothes the nervous system; alleviates urinary disorders; and improves elimination. Upon inverting the body, blood flows easily to the organs, especially the liver. It is also a key pose for boosting the immune system and helps treat colds, throat problems, and sinus congestion.*

Caution: *If you have back or neck problems, osteoporosis, high blood pressure, or heart problems, seek the advice of an experienced teacher before practicing this pose or the variations that follow.*

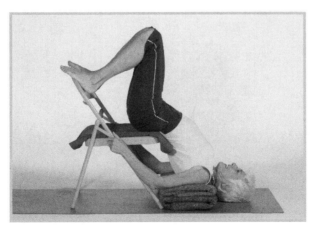

Lower your shoulders to the blanket, back of the head on the floor.

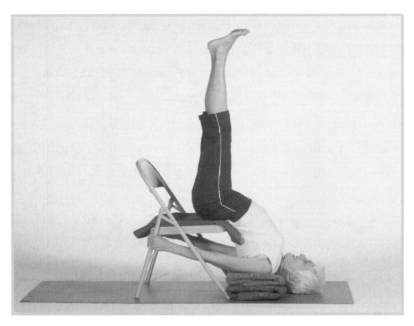

Shoulderstand with Chair, legs straight—the fountain of youth.

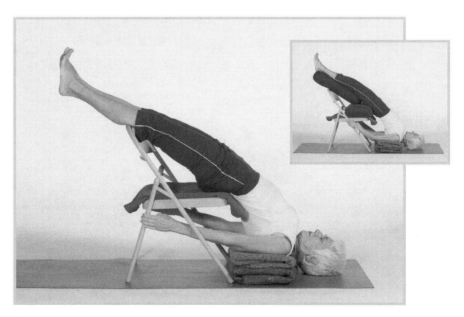

Shoulderstand with a Chair, sacrum on the edge of the chair seat.

Supported Half Plow Pose with a Chair
(Ardha Halasana)

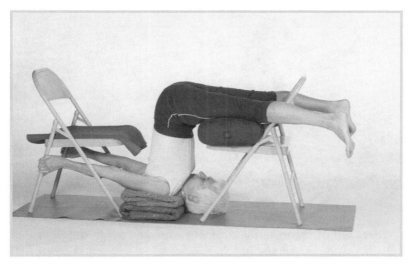

Half Plow Pose, active variation with the legs supported by a bolster placed on the chair seat.

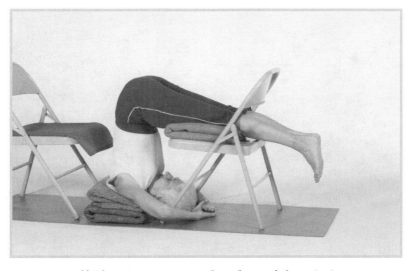

Half Plow Pose, arms relaxed, restful variation.

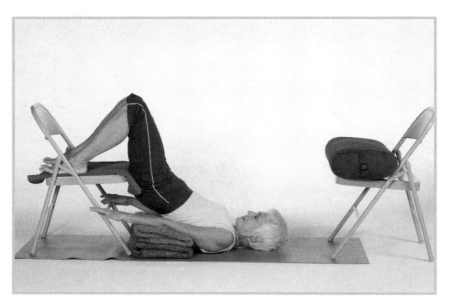

Come out of the pose by lowering your bottom to the floor and sliding your shoulders off the blanket.

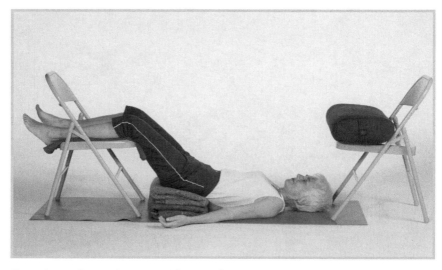

Rest for a few minutes with your legs on the chair seat, shoulders off the blanket.

Supported Half Plow Pose

This pose follows Supported Shoulderstand or can be practiced on its own. The legs are supported by the chair seat, allowing your body to relax completely while your organs invert.

- Depending on your height and flexibility, place two or three folded blankets on the chair seat so that your spine is extended in the pose. As in Shoulderstand, the shoulders are supported by two or three folded blankets placed near the legs of the chair. Lie with your shoulders on the blankets and your head under the chair seat.

- Bend your knees to your chest, and swing your legs over your head.

- Move your bottom toward your feet so that your thighs completely rest on the chair seat.

- Relax your arms back, palms facing up. Your teacher can show you how to make this healing pose truly comfortable.

Supported Shoulderstand and Supported Half Plow Pose should be practiced before Supported Legs Up the Wall Pose. It is extra rejuvenating to practice all three of these poses. Since Supported Legs Up the Wall Pose is completely passive, it is practiced after Supported Shoulderstand and Half Plow.

Benefits: *This pose is deeply relaxing for the mind and nervous system.*

JUDITH HANSON LASATER

Why Restorative Yoga Is Important as We Age

*J*udith Hanson Lasater, Ph.D, P.T., is the author of six books, including Relax and Renew: Restful Yoga for Stressful Times. *After
the death of her twin brother, she practiced restorative poses every day
for a year to help her with the grieving process. Restorative yoga is helpful for both the person who needs care and the caregiver. Judith gives
sound advice to the caregivers of the world: It is imperative that we take
care of ourselves, otherwise life's stresses will make us unable to care for
those who depend on us. Practicing restorative yoga releases us from
chronic stress and mitigates its debilitating effects.*

We work very hard most days, and while we may take time to sleep, we
rarely take time to rest deeply. Restorative yoga poses are special poses that
use blankets and bolsters to support the body and thus help us to relax and
rest deeply and completely.

During deep relaxation all the organ systems of the body are allowed to
rest. Measurable results of relaxation are the reduction of blood pressure
and the improvement of immune function, as well as improvement in
digestion, elimination, and the reduction of muscle tension and generalized
fatigue. Additionally there is promising indication that shows reduction in
serum triglycerides and "bad" cholesterol and some stabilization in blood-
sugar levels.

Restorative poses are simple, satisfying, and pleasant to practice. But the benefits are profound, whether we are ill or just "stressed out." Learning to give ourselves the gift of twenty minutes of quiet relaxation and reflection each day is one of the most powerful things we can do to improve our health.

As we age, stress accumulates in the body: We experience increased stress on our joints, on the heart, and on the lungs and liver, among other organs. The practice of restorative yoga not only helps the general health of the body; it also gives us a time of deep introspection and stillness, so necessary in today's outer-directed, overstimulated world.

Learning to trust the process of letting go in a daily restorative practice can teach us the joy of letting go of our hurts, our fears, and, when the time comes, our very lives.

One of the things I like about yoga
is its dignity. The more we submit ourselves to
the poses, surrender to the stressless discipline,
the more we can focus—the more
we are our true selves.

Betty Hodges,
79-year-old beginner

CHAPTER 12

The Last Asana

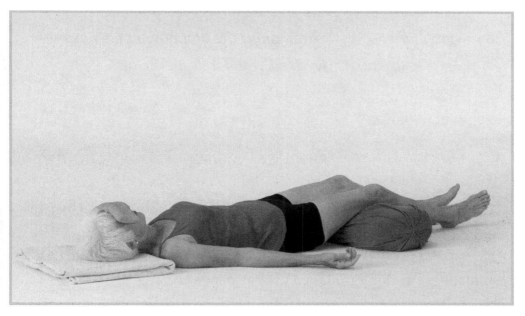

Savasana, *Corpse Pose.*

Death cuts you off with a very, very,
very sharp razor from your attachments, from
your gods, from your superstitions, from your desire
for comfort. . . . So how can I find out, actually,
not theoretically, what it means to die? It means to be
totally free, to be totally unattached to everything that man
has put together, or what you have put together . . .
totally free. . . . While you are living, every moment you
are dying, so that throughout life you are not attached
to anything. *That is what death means.*

J. Krishnamurti,
public talk, January 1, 1986,
six weeks before his death

Our yoga practice ends with *Savasana*, the Corpse Pose. In *Savasana*, we learn the art of letting go. The body lies as still and motionless as a corpse, the eyes closed, completely relaxed and at peace.

To understand *Savasana*, we begin with the fundamental yoga principle of *Ahimsa*, which means the recognition that all of life is sacred. *Ahimsa* entails an attitude of reverence toward all living beings. Out of our reverence for life, for example, we refrain from consuming sentient beings for our food if at all possible. *Ahimsa* is more than just kindness, although it includes that. *Ahimsa* is a dynamic principle that informs the quality of our action at every level.

Indeed, it is out of a spirit of *Ahimsa* that we do yoga at all, for we wish to cultivate and enhance the life force in ourselves, as well as in all other beings. Yoga practice is the expression of *Ahimsa* toward the health of our own body.

Savasana

In *Savasana*, we do not welcome death or wish to hasten its arrival. Nevertheless, we realize that its time will come. When that moment arrives, will we be ready? As the famous yogi William Shakespeare asked in *Hamlet*, can we "shuffle off this mortal coil" and face the unknown without fear and without regret?

Yoga teaches that we cannot be ready for death as long as we remain psychologically attached to the things of this world. In *Savasana*, we practice the art of releasing ourselves from our attachments and letting go.

Ahimsa and *Savasana* are not opposed to one another, but they do represent complementary principles. They are yin and yang to one another, moving in different directions but inseparable. There cannot be death without life—obviously. But it is equally true, though not so obvious, that there cannot be life without death.

Yoga teaches us to face death calmly, with equanimity, because we have already faced it and explored its implications while we are healthy and still have all our faculties. And because we have faced death we are moved even more strongly to practice *Ahimsa* as long as we remain here on this earthly plane.

Ahimsa (Nonviolence)

The great yoga masters through the ages have urged us to consider all aspects of our lives and to revere all living things.

Yoga addresses the ethical life through a whole range of practices that encourage us to live in harmony with nature, which includes how we treat animals. The practice of yoga is rooted in the principle of *ahimsa*, nonviolence and reverence for all life.

The great yoga masters teach that the yogi believes that every creature has as much right to live as he has. He believes he is born to help others, and he looks upon creation with the eyes of love. Yogis know that one's life is linked inextricably with other living things. A complete, holistic yoga practice encompasses a way of life that addresses the harm we inflict on all living things.

The influence of this asana on the body and the mind— from relaxation, to surrender, to death, and even after death—is incredible. If you do not want to be a living corpse, then the purpose of life has to be established. If you want to be an active participant in your life and not a parasite, then the dynamic interdependence between life and death has to be recognized, and the two have to meet in directed and concentrated interaction.

Swami Sivananda Radha,
Hatha Yoga: The Hidden Language

The Art of Deep Relaxation

In her workshops and writings on restorative yoga, Judith Hanson Lasater teaches the importance of a formal relaxation period of fifteen to thirty minutes per day, every day, in *Savasana*. Physiologically, it takes at least fifteen minutes before we can withdraw from the external sensations of the outer world.

If we lie still long enough in *Savasana*, we gradually discover the stages or levels of relaxation. In the first stage of *Savasana*, one becomes aware of the unrelenting activity of the brain, the constant noise and chatter of thoughts, feelings, and muscular fidgeting. But if the body remains still, the activity of the brain slows, blood pressure drops, breathing and heart rate slow.

In *Savasana* we create space for the mind and body to slowly unwind, to loosen their grip, to release tension, and to relax. In the beginning, *Savasana* may simply feel like a welcome rest. We may sink or wander in and out of a sleep state, especially if we are sleep deprived. With practice we remain aware and move into the deeper stages of *Savasana* where there is a palpable shift in the body and mind. The outer world drifts away, and we experience divine rest.

In Shavasana, *relaxation is the first*
attempt to surrender, to let go. As the mind follows
the flow of the breath, the ripples of the mental
lake slowly subside. With continued practice,
the senses are gradually withdrawn and become still.
Passion, egocentricity, self-importance are, for
the moment, put to rest. Sufficient rest allows the
body to recuperate from the driving forces of
the emotions and the ambitions of the mind.
The benefits—physically, mentally, emotionally—
are profound. In that state of peace and quiet
and inner harmony, one can perceive a vision of the
Light that is present in both life and death.

Swami Sivananda Radha,
Hatha Yoga: The Hidden Language

The Practice of *Savasana*

Ideally, *Savasana* is practiced in a quiet place where we will
not be disturbed. The practice can be as simple as lying on the
floor in a quiet place without any props, or with the support
of a bolster, eye bag, blankets, or other props arranged to
allow the experience of ever-deeper levels of relaxation.

Savasana *I: Deep Relaxation (Corpse) Pose*

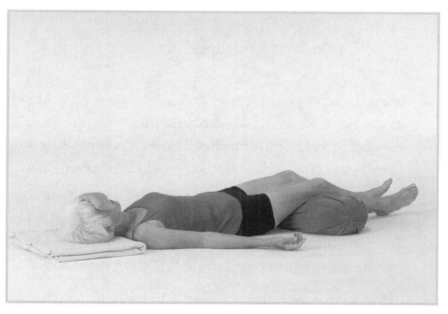

Savasana *with bolster under knees, eye bag over eyes, to relax the mind.*

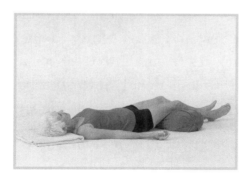

Savasana *on floor, bolster under knees, to relax the lower back.*

In *Savasana*, the body resides symmetrically on the floor, with the palms turned up, arms equidistant from the midline of the body.

- Sit on the floor with the upper body and legs in a straight line.

- Lean back on your elbows and lower your back slowly to the floor. Place a folded blanket under your head if needed to keep your forehead and chin level. Center your head, chin in line with the center of your chest.

- Allow your mouth to feel as if you are about to smile so your throat, jaw, and face muscles soften and relax. The weight of an eye bag over your eyes quiets the movement of your eyes and helps the brain to relax.

- Extend your legs and feet and allow them to fall evenly away from the midline.

- As you lie still, let your mind follow the peaceful flow of your breath. Be aware of the beating of your heart and allow the chest and heart center to open and relax. Allow your eyes to sink into their sockets, to turn inward and to look deeply into your body. Allow your body to release and sink toward the Earth.

- *Stay in the pose for fifteen minutes.*

- When you feel ready to sit up, bend your knees and turn to your side for a few breaths; use your hands to press the floor as you sit up.

Like other yoga poses, *Savasana* requires that your body be in alignment. When you attend a yoga class, your teacher has an aerial view of your body and checks to see that you are allowing the left and right sides of your body to relax evenly into the floor. If you are practicing this pose on your own, you will benefit more from the pose if a friend who practices yoga checks your position. It may take some time to adjust and align your posture. Just as the wall gives you feedback about your posture when standing upright, observe the way each part of your body rests on the floor.

If lying with your legs straight feels uncomfortable in your lower back, place a folded blanket or bolster under your knees. Some people feel more comfortable with their lower legs supported on a chair.

A ten-pound sandbag across the pelvis, or a sandbag over the top of each thigh, helps the body sink into the floor and adds immeasurably to the depth of relaxation.

Trust the process of *Savasana*. When we lie still, we are practicing what yogis refer to as "deliberate stillness." We give the mind and body a chance to integrate the events of our Life and let go of the past. Consciously practicing the art of letting go may help prepare us for the inevitable transition from life to death.

Savasana II: *Supported Deep Relaxation (Corpse) Pose*

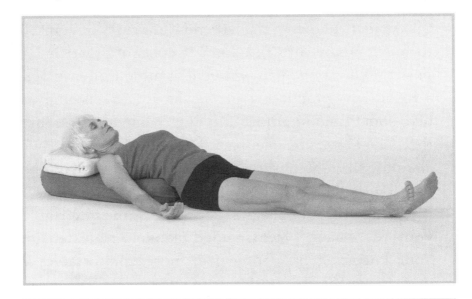

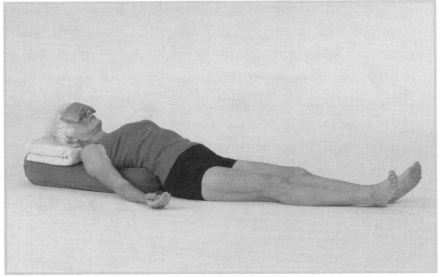

*Supported **Savasana**, bolster under back, folded blanket under head, eye bag over eyes. Relaxing with the back supported makes breathing easier and rests the heart.*

- Sit in front of a bolster (or two or three blankets folded lengthwise) with one or two folded blankets at the top of the bolster to create a comfortable support for your head and neck. The edge of the bolster should touch your tailbone. Before lying back, look down the front of your body, and see if your upper body and lower body are centered so that the line formed by the nose, chin, center of your chest, navel, and pubic bone extends directly toward a center point between your heels.

- Center your spine on the bolster. You may have to experiment with the height of the blanket under your head so that it feels truly comfortable. Your forehead should be higher than your chin and should not drop back.

- Place an eye bag over your eyes. Relax your arms on the floor with your hands about a foot from your hips. Turn your palms up, and stretch your fingers outward, turning your thumbs toward the floor. Allow your arms and hands to soften and relax. Allow your legs and feet to relax and fall away from the midline. Your body should feel supremely comfortable, supported by the bolster, blankets, and floor.

- If you feel discomfort in your back, try repositioning your back on the bolster—you may be too high or too low on the bolster. If you still feel strain, decrease the height under your back, or place a folded blanket under your bottom.

Benefits: *Supporting the length of your spine and back of the head opens the chest and allows the breath to flow freely. A teacher can*

INSTRUCTIONS

show you various ways to arrange stacks of blankets to open the chest, which is particularly beneficial for heart and respiratory problems. Opening the chest is an antidote to depression and helps remove physical, mental, and emotional fatigue.

Savasana relaxes the body, soothes the nervous system, lowers blood pressure and heart rate, and brings a sense of peace to the mind. It helps relieve migraine and stress-related headaches and can be helpful for insomnia. If you have trouble sleeping, practice this pose before going to bed or when you have difficulty falling back to sleep.

Yoga Prepares Us for Life's Greatest Journey

My feelings about death changed dramatically 25 years ago with my first yoga class. After guiding me through the first half of the primary series of Ashtanga Yoga, my teacher asked me to lie down and then covered me with a blanket. As I lay there on the floor I felt myself settling into a relaxed state listening to the Ujjayi breathing of the other students and watching the candlelight flickering on the walls. Gradually I began to feel first my body, and then my mind let go as I descended deeper into stillness. In that stillness I experienced a sense of calm, spacious awareness that felt like home—a home that was very familiar even though it hadn't been visited in some time. A great sense of comfort and reassurance came over me, knowing that deep within myself was this bedrock of being that felt clear, open, and endless.

Tim Miller,
"How Yoga Can Prepare Us for Death," www.yogajournal.com.

SHIRLEY DAVENTRY FRENCH
Do Not Waste the Gift of Old Age

S hirley is a direct student of B. K. S. Iyengar and one of North America's most experienced teachers of the Iyengar method of yoga. She has been teaching in Victoria and throughout Canada for over thirty years and gives workshops nationally and internationally. She has also studied extensively with Swami Sivananda Radha at Yasodhara Ashram, British Columbia.

When I celebrated my seventieth birthday, along with the congratulations I received many comments along the lines of "Oh no, you can't be! It isn't possible!" Even before this landmark, if ever I referred to myself as old, this was met with a quick disclaimer: "Oh you're not old!" Sometimes I would take the time to point out that if you took my age and doubled it you would reach a figure well beyond the current limit of human life, so I could hardly be called middle-aged. Such logic would generally produce another quick response: "Well, you don't look old!"

Getting old is such a taboo topic in North America. Most people want to get away from it as quickly as possible. A few years ago I had what I thought was a good idea: to offer a course about growing old. I had the temerity (or stupidity if I had wanted it to be a financial success) to call it just that: *Growing Old.* I did make a concession toward optimism by adding the subheading *A Time of Growth* and explaining that in the Eastern spiritual tradition old age is viewed as a gift of time to focus on one's own spiritual development.

Women of sixty years of age or older who wanted to explore their spiritual goals within the framework of yogic teachings were invited to join in discussions led by myself and a fellow yoga teacher, Jessica Sluymer. The course would provide an opportunity [for participants] to talk about their aging without being dismissed or cut off with pleasantries and to discover how yoga can help bring meaning and value to this stage of life.

The idea for this course emerged from Jessica and from my own explorations and concretized in a conversation we had over lunch one day about our own aging process. "We are getting older," I announced sagaciously. "We are old!" Jessica (who is the same age as me) responded, and we both burst out laughing.

We did not have huge expectations that this would be a very popular course, and we were right. Several of the students from my seniors class came up to me and said that when I offered a class called *Growing Younger* then they would be interested. This may have been said partly in jest, but in our culture it is common to deny and attempt to hide our aging and consequently waste this gift that longevity has earned. In the end, there were five of us, including the two teachers. One of the women was dying, which brought a sobriety and immediacy to these sessions.

Our inevitable demise has to be faced sooner or later, but most of us live our lives as if it will be later. As the American writer William Saroyan is reputed to have said when he was dying, "I knew everyone had to die, but somehow I thought an exception would be made in my case!"

My husband has told me about patients of his, in their eighties or nineties, who were still denying their mortality. In fact, one patient of his, whom he had looked after for many years, discharged Derek as his doctor when he was close to a hundred years old because he wanted a doctor who would make him feel better. He showed no gratitude at all for the help he had received through many medical crises in which he had come close to death, or for the frequent and regular house calls at all times of day. He was, of course, quite within his rights to change doctors, but his new doctor was also unable to stem the tide of time, and this man died shortly thereafter.

We will either grow old or die young or in midlife. We do not have a lot of choice. If we are fortunate enough to live to be old, the quality of that life as it draws to its close is to a very large extent up to us.

LEIGH MILNE
Why Do We Do Yoga?

*W*hile I was writing this book, Leigh Milne, whose story appears in Chapter 10, shared this anecdote with me about Father Joe. Father Joe is a senior teacher who has worked closely with B. K. S. Iyengar for many years. He spent over twenty years working beside Mother Teresa. He combines yoga and meditation to support people living with addictions, AIDS, and HIV.

A fellow yogi told me a story about a Father Joe Pereira workshop held in Toronto. During the lunch break Father Joe was asked "Why do we do yoga?" His reply was "To prepare for death." This was more than the student was prepared for, and he did not return to the workshop that afternoon.

Death is not a matter that most of us spend much time considering, especially when we are younger. In fact, our culture would consider us morbid if we did. Mr. Iyengar has said that he now practices in preparation to meet God. At his eighty-fourth birthday celebration he said, "You must look deep into your Self, which is like a dark cave." One meaning for the word *Guru* is "A teacher who leads from darkness into light." Yoga can lead us through that darkness.

I write this while my father is dying. He is in the last stages of his cancer, lying in a hospital bed in a sunny room on a special wing, with two other men, also there to die. Most of the time my dad is quiet, even while awake, and although he is not a yogi or a religious man, I wonder if, in the silence of these last days, he has been inside his cave and found something more than darkness there. *"Tada drashtuh svarupe avasthanam."* ("Then, the seer dwells in his/her own true splendor.") (I.III *Yoga Sutras*).

I visit daily, sit, and hold his hand for hours—a seated meditation. I've noticed how difficult it is for other visitors to be still, how uncomfortable they are to just be in the present moment, in the presence of my father's dying. This is something I can do. It is my yoga.

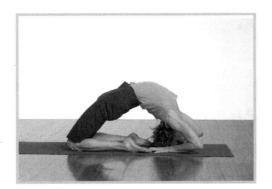

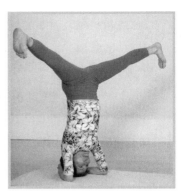

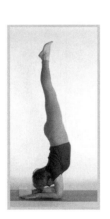

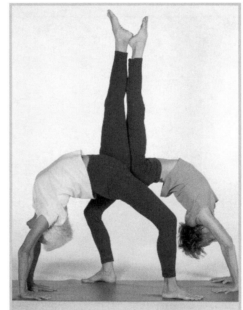

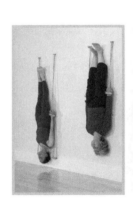

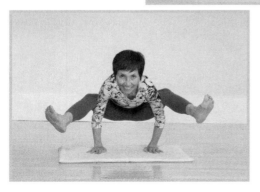

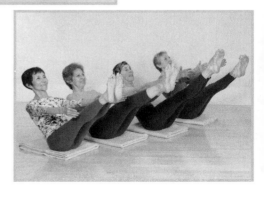

MEET THE MODELS

*In everyone's life, at some time, our inner fire
goes out. It is then burst into flame by an encounter
with another human being. We should all be thankful
for those people who rekindle the inner spirit.*

Albert Schweitzer, philosopher,
physician, author, and karma yogi

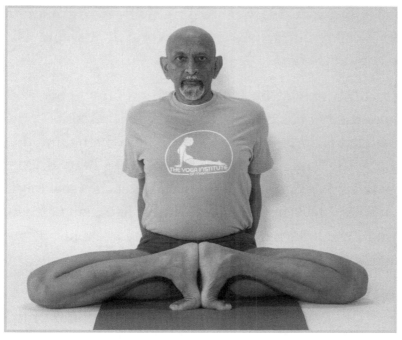

Ramanand Patel in an advanced seated pose known as Root Chakra Pose,
Mulabandhasana. *Seated poses calm the mind and are vital to the health of
all the systems of the body.*

Ramanand Patel is in his mid-sixties. He was initiated into yoga practice by his father at the age of twelve. He studied with many different teachers and became a student of B. K. S. Iyengar in 1968. He is a founding member of the Iyengar Yoga Teacher Training Institute of San Francisco, where he is known as "the teacher's teacher." He is well-known as an innovator in the use of props and for working with students who have special needs. He combines his technical expertise with knowledge of Vedanta philosophy. Ramanand has a special interest in the effects of sound on yoga practice and offers workshops in this subject with musician Pandit Mukesh Desai. He conducts teacher-training seminars throughout the world. To find out where in the world Ramanand is, visit www.yogirama.com.

Betty Eiler arrived on Planet Earth on November 22, 1934. Ramanand Patel has been her primary teacher since 1984. She has traveled to India to study with B. K. S. Iyengar and Geeta Iyengar at the Ramamani Memorial Institute. Betty divides her time between Mexico and California. She teaches several classes a week when she is in the United States. To e-mail Betty for her teaching schedule, write to bettyme@comcast.net. For more about Betty, read her story on page 26.

Barbara Wiechmann was born on March 23, 1943, in Fayetteville, Arkansas. She has been studying and practicing yoga for over thirty years. In 1987, she studied with B. K. S. Iyengar at the Ramamani Iyengar Memorial Institute in Pune, where she and Betty Eiler first met. Her primary teachers are Judith Hanson Lasater and Ramanand Patel at the Iyengar

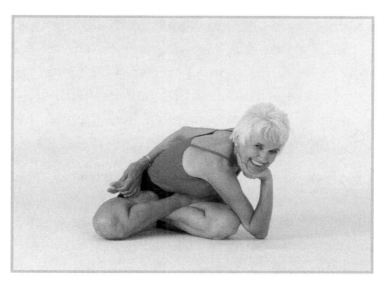

Betty Eiler in a Lotus Pose variation.

Yoga Institute in San Francisco, where she acquired her yoga teacher certification. She continues to study regularly with Ramanand Patel. She has taught yoga classes in San Francisco for over two decades. She also teaches at the Bija Yoga Center in San Francisco, where many of the photographs in this book were taken.

Barbara wore many hats during the photo sessions for this book. Besides being an inspiring, ageless yoga model, she also assisted Jim at all the shoots. She demonstrated poses and adjusted the other models, helped set up the yoga room, brought props and carried equipment, and assisted with many other details essential to a good photo shoot. Barbara's story on how she discovered yoga appears on page 34. For information about Barbara's classes at the Bija Yoga Studio visit www.bijayoga.com. To e-mail Barbara for her class schedule, write to barbara@c255.ucsf.edu.

Toni Montez was born on March 28, 1927. She was on the staff of the Institute for Yoga Teacher Education (now the Iyengar Yoga Institute of San Francisco) for many years and was one of my first teachers. She has studied with B. K. S. Iyengar in India and with other teachers around the world. Her story appears on page 198.

Judith Alper has been practicing Iyengar-style yoga since 1975 and began teaching in 1978. She also practices Vipassana Meditation. As a retired attorney, she recently returned to teaching yoga and completed the Advanced Studies Program at the Yoga Room in Berkeley. While her primary teacher over the years has been Donald Moyer (author of *Yoga: Awakening the Inner Body*) at the Yoga Room in Berkeley, California, she has also benefited greatly from studying with Mary Lou Weprin, Jerry Byrd, Judith Hanson Lasater (whose writing appears in Chapter 11), Ramanand Patel and Rama Jyoti Vernon. She credits yoga with helping her to survive both law school and cancer and with keeping her body active and flexible into her seventh decade. Photos of Judith practicing and teaching her octogenarian student Lewis Perry can be seen in Chapters 3, 8, and 10. For information about Judith's classes at the Berkeley Yoga Center, visit www.Berkeleyyoga.com. To e-mail Judith for her class schedule, write to judithalper@sbcglobal.net.

Lewis Perry was born October 30, 1922. He is eighty-three years old and has been taking a yoga class once a week for about three years. He studies with Judith Alper and feels that his flexibility is improved and that his ability to move around and his enjoyment of life are greatly enhanced by yoga.

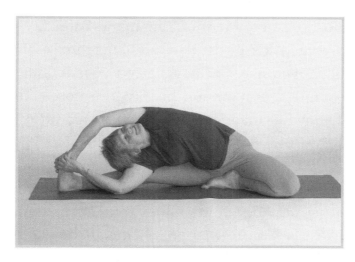

Judith Alper in Revolved Head to Knee Pose, **Parivritta Janusirsasana,** *a delicious revolved seated pose that gives a rejuvenating stretch to the hips, shoulders, and back.*

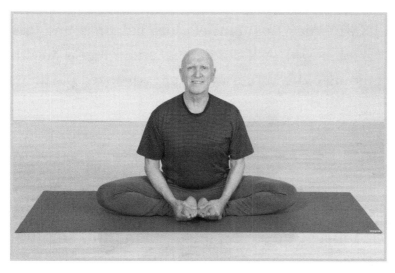

Olney Fortier demonstrates Bound-Angle Pose, **Baddha Konasana.** *When he first began practicing, he sat on two folded blankets to lengthen the back of his body and to help keep the front of his body open.*

Olney Fortier is a student of Ramanand Patel. So far Olney has not divulged his birth date, but he promises he is well qualified for "over sixty." Olney started yoga a few years ago with hip openers, still among his favorite poses. To see the progress Olney has made in his favorite seated poses—Seated Bound-Angle Pose, *Baddha Konasana,* and Seated Wide-Angle Pose, *Upavistha Konasana*—and how Ramanand teaches him these poses, see Chapter 10. After watching Betty Eiler practicing *Hanumanasana,* Yoga Splits, Olney told me that in ten years, when I write *The New Yoga for People Over 70,* he wants to do a photo with him and Betty doing the splits together. With his dedication and daily practice, I believe he will do it!

Tsuneko Hellerstein, age seventy-nine, has practiced yoga on her own for many years and is in her second year of teacher training at the Iyengar Yoga Institute of San Francisco. Her teachers include Kathy Alef, Nora Burnett, Joe Nadzunas, and Jaki Nett. Jaki is a *Yoga Journal* "Ask the Expert" editor and is an expert in safely guiding older bodies into more advanced positions.

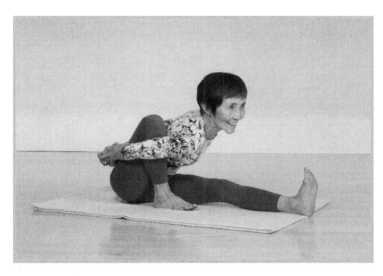

*Seventy-nine-year-old Tsuneko Hellerstein in a seated pose, **Marichyasana I**, named after the Indian sage Marici. This is a complex pose in which the body first twists to the side and then bends forward.*

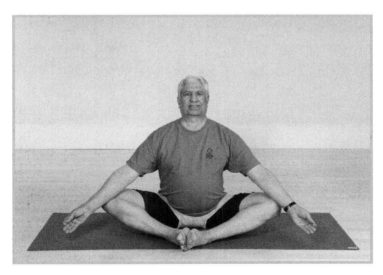

*Parminder Singh Ghuman, age sixty-eight, sits in Bound-Angle Pose, **Baddha Konasana**. A long stay in this pose, when practiced with quiet breathing, helps to induce a peaceful, meditative frame of mind.*

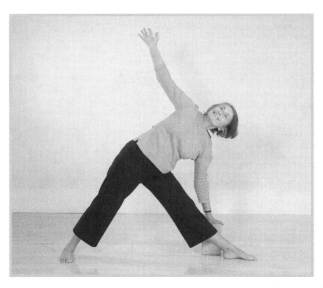

Lillian Cartwright, age seventy-three, enjoys stretching in Extended Triangle Pose, **Trikonasana,** *one of the essential poses for safely removing stiffness in all parts of the body.*

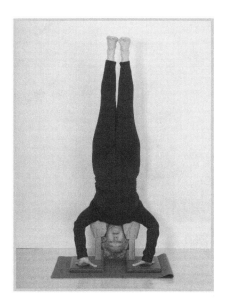

Neti Fredericks, in her late sixties, demonstrates a safe way to reverse gravity by turning herself upside down using the Headstander, a yoga prop.

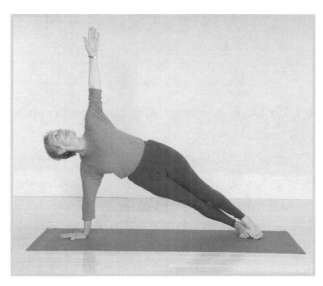

Margaret Ghuman, age sixty-six, strengthens her arms and upper body in Plank Pose with one arm up, **Vasisthasana.**

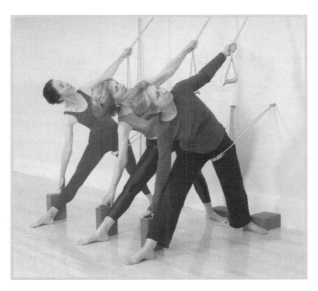

Josefina Vigne, age seventy-nine, and Karen Brelin and Judy Goldhalft, in their mid-sixties, practice Extended Triangle Pose, **Utthita Trikonasana,** *holding onto the wall rope with the upper hand, to improve balance, increase flexibility, and maintain healthy alignment of the spine.*

MEET THE PHOTOGRAPHER
AND HIS ASSISTANT

Jim Jacobs, Ph.D., is a fine art and commercial photographer, as well as a clinical psychologist, in Berkeley, California. He studied photography at the San Francisco Art Institute. One of his projects is photographing people exhibiting beauty, grace, and character in midlife and beyond. Working with yoga practitioners over sixty is part of this project. Jim was the lead photographer for *The New Yoga for People Over 50*. His credits include photographs in *Yoga Journal*, *Yoga Journal* calendars, and other yoga publications. A serious Iyengar yoga practitioner himself for over twenty years, Jim is a longtime student of Ramanand Patel and Melinda Perlee. Born in 1941, his yoga story appears on page 154.

For information about Jim Jacobs Photography, visit www.jimjacobsphotography.com or write to jim@jimjacobsphotography.com.

Alex Jacobs Hirth, Jim Jacobs's thirteen-year-old son, has assisted on every photography shoot for this book. Jim says, "I don't know what I would have done without him, particularly in loading and setting up heavy, complicated equipment. He has a good eye and an inventive mind, so I frequently take his suggestions." Thanks to Alex's assistance, Jim was able to be both the photographer and one of the models for some photos in this book. Jim set up those shots and Alex triggered the shutter.

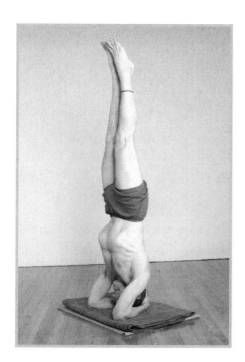 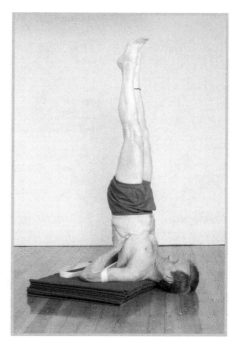

Jim Jacobs demonstrates Headstand, **Sirsasana,** *and* **Shoulderstand, Salamba Sarvangasana,** *known as the Two Pillars, the King and the Queen, or the Father and Mother of Yoga.*

According to his father, Alex's first word was *yoga.* "I swear he said it at nine months when I was in Plow Pose." At four years old, Alex "took pictures" with his improvised camera and tripod: a forked stick. He first attended his father's yoga photo shoots when he was five.

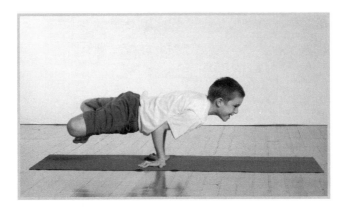

Alex Jacobs Hirth enjoys practicing a variation of the Peacock Pose with the legs in Full Lotus Pose, known as **Padma Mayurasana**. *Here he is practicing with Barbara Wiechmann, an example of "ageless yoga."*

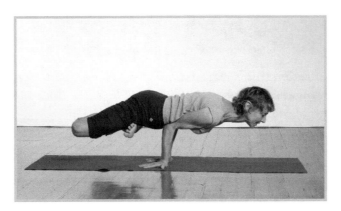

Barbara Wiechmann practicing the Peacock Pose with Alex Jacobs Hirth.

APPENDIX A

Yoga for Stroke Survivors

S troke is the leading cause of adult disability in the United States. According to the U.S. Centers for Disease Control, one American suffers a stroke every forty-five seconds. Each year, more than 700,000 people have a stroke; about two-thirds of them are age sixty and older.

A stroke occurs when the brain is deprived of blood. This can happen when a blood vessel is ruptured or is blocked by a clot. The lack of oxygen damages or kills brain cells and disrupts functions controlled by the affected part of the brain. Because blood brings vital oxygen and nutrients to the brain, this deprivation can have devastating effects if not treated immediately.

Most people who survive a stroke require therapy to restore function, and most of them also report impaired health status because of a reduced level of activity. The practice of yoga can play a vital role in their recovery processes.

Stroke Guidelines for Teachers

Many of the guidelines presented throughout this book are helpful for working with students who have survived a stroke. The difficulties faced by stroke victims vary widely. Two common problems after a stroke are difficulty with balance (associated with increased risk for falls) and one-sided weakness affecting an arm or leg or both.

If the student is able to move easily (or with minimal assistance) from a chair to the floor, consider beginning the yoga session lying on the back, with adequate support under the head so that the forehead is higher than the chin. Be extra careful that the head does not tilt back. If a student feels dizzy when lying down, elevate the head more to see if the dizziness goes away promptly.

Many poses can be practiced lying on the floor and even in bed. Support the body with folded blankets, bolsters, and sandbags as needed. Chairs, walls, ropes, the yoga horse, and other props can all be used to adapt yoga to the needs of the person with stroke and disabilities.

A stroke survivor will likely have serious underlying medical problems, such as high blood pressure, heart disease, or glaucoma. For this reason, inversions and variations of inversions are generally avoided and should only be practiced under the supervision of a knowledgeable teacher. Practice supported lying-down poses instead.

Modify Standing Forward Bend Poses by practicing with the body parallel to the floor and with the hands on a wall or other sturdy level surface. In general, avoid poses where the head is below the waist. As strength and balance improve, students can begin to practice basic standing poses with their backs against a wall and their bottom hands on the back of a chair or chair seat, depending on their flexibility (see Chapter 3). Students should keep their heads in a neutral position and focus on lengthening their necks.

Stroke survivors can benefit immensely from learning to gently deepen their breathing without strain. Observing and regulating the flow of the breath is calming and helps bring the mind and body into the present moment. Encourage the student to sit or lie down with the chest open, using props as needed to prevent slouching. A bolster or a slender, firm pillow, known as a *pranayama bolster* or *breathing bolster*, can be used to support the length of the spine and back of the head and to maintain healthy, open posture when sitting in a chair or wheelchair. Blankets and other firm pillows can also be used to help stroke survivors relearn and maintain good posture.

Stroke brings up many difficult issues, including anxiety, grief over lost ability, and uncertainty about recovery and what it means to become dependent on the care of other people. Stroke is also connected to conscious dying and the right to choose to die before one's mental capacities are affected. Many years ago, I helped a woman who had a stroke and lost control of some of her bodily functions. She did not want to enter a nursing home and risk declining to a point where she did not know where she was or who she was. She chose instead to stop eating so she could leave her body consciously.

I highly recommend consulting with a teacher or physical therapist who has experience working with stroke patients.

(See Appendix C for organizations that may be able to help you find someone in your area.) Many teachers develop an interest in working with people with stroke after a friend or family member has a stroke. Learn by working with someone one-on-one before teaching a group.

Many books and videos are available on therapeutic applications of yoga and may be helpful, even if they do not focus specifically on stroke recovery. The following websites, books and videos provide an excellent starting place.

Resources for Yoga, Stroke, and Disabilities

Bell, Baxter, M.D. "Yoga for Stroke Survivors," *Yoga Journal*. Retrieved in 2006 at yogajournal.com/practice/967_1.cfm. Dr. Bell teaches yoga classes in northern California and lectures to healthcare professionals around the country. He integrates the therapeutic applications of yoga with Western medicine. His newsletters and videos can be found at www.bellyoga.info.

Bell, Lorna, R.N., and Eudora Seyfer. *Gentle Yoga for People with Arthritis, Stroke Damage, Multiple Sclerosis or People in Wheelchairs*. Berkley, CA: Celestial Arts, 1987.

Biermann, June, and Barbara Toohey. *The Stroke Book: A Guide to Life After Stroke for Survivors and Those Who Care for Them*. New York: Tarcher/Penguin, 2005.

Dickman, Carol. *Bedtop Yoga, Chair Yoga*, Videos for Seniors. Yoga audiotapes for the blind and visually impaired. www.yogaeze.com; carol@stretch.com.

Dworkis, Sam. *Recovery Yoga: A Practical Guide for Chronically Ill, Injured, and Post-Operative People*. New York: Three Rivers Press, 1997. www.extensionyoga.com.

Fishman, Loren Martin, M.D., and Eric Small. *Yoga and Multiple Sclerosis: A Journey to Health and Healing*. New York: Demos Medical Publishing, 2006. A video, articles, and related links are available at www.yogaMS.com.

Newborn, Barbara. *Return to Ithaca: A Young Woman's Triumph Over the Disabilities of a Severe Stroke*. Rockport, MA: Element Books, 1997. Barbara Newborn teaches yoga for the severely disabled. She is currently the chief of staff of the National Stroke and Quality of Life Medical Education Institute at Columbia Presbyterian Medical Center in New York. Her book provides a brief appendix that gives relevant facts about the occurrence, clinical features, and economic costs of stroke, as well as a list of resources available for stroke patients and their families. (813) 831-1598; gardensofyoga.com; barbnewborn@yahoo.com.

Ram Dass. *Fierce Grace*. Zeitgeist Films, 2003. This documentary about Ram Dass chronicles his struggle to reconcile his message of unconditional love and acceptance with the anger and frustration he feels about the stroke that left half of his body paralyzed.

Sanford, Matthew. *Waking: A Memoir of Transcendence*. Emmaus, PA: Rodale Books, 2006. Matthew will speak to any audience interested in the relationship between mind–body integration and disability. (952) 484-9791; www.matthewsanford.com; mbsolutions@earthlink.net.

Small, Eric. *See* Fishman, Loren Martin.

Zwick, Dalia, P.T. Rehabyoga.com is an educational website designed to communicate the benefits of yoga for people in physical therapy, their caregivers, and their therapists. Highly recommended for those who are teaching yoga to stroke survivors. www.rehabyoga.com. E-mail: info@rehabyoga.com.

Note: *See Appendix C for additional resources that may be helpful for those recovering from a stroke.*

APPENDIX B

Yoga and Memory Loss

My first yoga teacher told me that she discovered yoga about the time she put her mother and mother-in-law in a rest home. In the course of teaching me how to practice Headstand, she explained, "The agony of taking them to a rest home after they were senile made a profound impression on me. I began to consider that perhaps I could hold back or even prevent senility by increasing the flow of blood to my brain through the inverted postures."

One of the areas that could benefit the most from a collaboration between medical research and yoga is memory loss. Yogis, including doctors who practice yoga, have long speculated that the practice of Headstand and other inverted poses can play an important role in keeping the brain sharp.

Two of the comments I hear frequently from my elderly students during and after class are "I can think better" and "My mind seems clearer." This may be anecdotal evidence, but it is certainly important to my students and to me, and it warrants further research.

Can Exercise Delay Alzheimer's Disease?

Studies demonstrate that seniors who engage in some form of exercise at least three days a week can cut their risk of developing Alzheimer's disease and other forms of dementia by as much as 30 to 40 percent.

Between 1994 and 2003, Dr. Eric B. Larson, director of the Group Health Cooperative's Center for Health Studies in Seattle, Washington, and his research team assessed the health, physical and mental function, and lifestyle characteristics of 1,740 men and women over the age of sixty-five.

All the people were members of a Seattle-based health maintenance organization. None had been diagnosed with dementia or were living in a nursing home at the start of the study.

Every two years, the researchers used examinations and in-person interviews to evaluate participants' weekly exercise routines; physical abilities such as walking, standing, balancing, and gripping; memory, attentiveness, and concentration skills; and smoking, drinking, and dietary supplement habits. Reporting in the *Annals of Internal Medicine* (January 16, 2006), the researchers noted that those who had been engaging in regular exercise at least three days a week when the study began had a 32 percent lower risk of developing dementia than those exercising less than three days a week.

The more frail a person is, the more he or she may benefit from exercise. According to the study, regular exercisers who had been evaluated as among the most physically weak at the start of the study experienced even more of a reduction in dementia risk.

Dr. Larson and his colleagues recommend further studies to explore how exercise can best improve circulation and oxygen delivery while reducing brain cell loss, which researchers suspect accounts for the resulting drop in dementia risk.

For more on Alzheimer's disease, see the National Institute of Aging website: www.nia.nih.gov.

APPENDIX C

Resources

I have included here many of the people, organizations, videos, and other sources of information consulted in the course of writing this book. Most of the websites listed here link to other sites that can help you find yoga teachers and centers in your area, as well as doctors and other health professionals that use yoga in their practices. This section also includes sources for yoga wall ropes, chairs, and other props recommended in this book.

Yoga with Suza Francina

Suza Francina, R.Y.T.
P.O. Box 1258
Ojai, CA 93024
(805) 646-4673
www.suzafrancina.com
SFrancina@aol.com

Yoga Teachers Featured in This Book

Judith Alper
www.Berkeleyyoga.com
judithalper@sbcglobal.net

Nora Burnett
www.noraburnett.com
nlburnett@earthlink.net

Sam Dworkis
Recovery Yoga
(561) 333-3690
www.extensionyoga.com
extensionyoga@yahoo.com

Betty Eiler
bettyme@comcast.net

Janice Freeman-Bell, R.Y.T.
Life Center, Cal State University, Sacramento
www.cdbaby.com/oconnellnfreeman
janice@surewest.net

Shirley Daventry French
Iyengar Yoga Centre of Victoria
202–919 Fort St., Victoria, BC, V8V 3K3 Canada
(250) 386-YOGA (9642)
www.iyengaryogacentre.ca
iyoga@telus.net

Carol Krucoff, R.Y.T.
www.healingmoves.com
healingmoves@aol.com

Judith Hanson Lasater, Ph.D., P.T.
www.judithlasater.com

Leigh A. Milne, R.M.T., R.Y.T., P.F.T.
www.yogamudra.com
leigh@yogamudra.com

A slide show of Leigh's study on the benefits of yoga for seniors can be viewed on her website.

Toni Montez
Tonimontez@aol.com

Ramanand Patel
1378 30th Ave.
San Francisco, CA 94122–1410
www.yogirama.com

Sandra Pleasants
sandrapleasants@msn.com

Felice Rhiannon
www.transformativeyoga.com
lotuses108@syv.com

Barbara Wiechmann
www.bijayoga.com
barbara@c255.ucsf.edu

Eleanor Williams
Eleanor@yoga.com

Finding a Teacher in Your Area

The organizations, directories, associations, and registries listed here can help you find a qualified teacher in your area. Most yoga centers offer introductory courses, level-one or beginner classes that may be suitable for all ages, including seniors. Others have special classes described as "Yoga 50+," "Yoga for Seniors," "Gentle Iyengar Yoga" or similar wording that indicates that the class considers the needs of older students. Some teachers state in their brochures that they have a "special interest in working with midlife and older students."

B. K. S. Iyengar's website
www.bksiyengar.com

The Green Yoga Association
www.GreenYoga.org
Studios@greenyoga.org

Offers resources for yoga studios to "green" their businesses. Their online newsletter has links to green studios, practitioners, and products, as well as eco-friendly yoga props. Healthy aging and the health of the planet are intimately connected.

International Association of Yoga Therapists (IAYT)
(928) 541-0004
www.iayt.org
mail@iayt.org

Here you can find teachers, therapists, doctors, and other health practitioners who utilize yoga in their practices. The IAYT website has links to extensive bibliographies that contain information on what yoga resources are available for a wide range of health and aging-related topics.

Iyengar Yoga Institute of San Francisco
(415) 753-0909
www.iyisf.org
info@iyisf.org

This is where I learned how to teach yoga to people at midlife and older!

Iyengar Yoga National Association of the United States
(800) 889-YOGA (9642)
www.iynaus.org

Iyengar Yoga Resources
International, comprehensive website for Iyengar yoga
www.iyengar-yoga.com

Julie Lawrence
Julie Lawrence Yoga Center
Portland, Oregon
www.jlyc.com

Gentle, slower-paced Iyengar yoga classes, ideal for seniors. Programs here are being studied by researchers at the Oregon Health & Science University.

Silver Age Yoga
Frank Iszak, Director, Founder
7968 Arjons Drive, Suite 213
San Diego, CA 92126
(858) 693-3110; toll free: (866) 751-0011
www.silverageyoga.org
silverageyoga@yahoo.com

Silver Age Yoga Community Outreach (SAYCO) is a nonprofit organization that trains teachers how to teach seniors and improve the lives of seniors by providing affordable yoga classes.

Yoga Alliance
Toll-free: (877) 964-2255
www.yogaalliance.org

Yoga Alliance registers both individual teachers and teacher training programs (schools) who have complied with educational standards established by the organization.

Yoga International Magazine
(800) 253-6243
www.yimag.org

Yoga Journal
(800) 600-9642
www.yogajournal.com
> Information on all aspects of yoga. Annual directory of teachers internationally.

Yoga Doctors, Yoga Therapists, and Yoga Therapy Centers

Baxter Bell, M.D.
(510) 681-4161
www.bellyoga.info
baxbellmd@hotmail.com

> Dr. Bell teaches yoga in northern California, nationally, and internationally. He integrates the therapeutic applications of yoga with Western medicine and lectures to healthcare professionals around the country. Newsletter and videos.

Roger Cole, Ph.D.
(858) 720-0076
www.yogadelmar.com
info@yogadelmar.com

> Roger Cole is a scientist, yoga teacher, and expert on sleep physiology. He teaches workshops nationally and internationally.

Gail Dubinsky, M.D.
www.rxyoga.com
> Specializes in yoga for repetitive stress injury. Videos available.

Dynamic Systems Rehabilitation Center
Matthew J. Taylor, P.T., Ph.D., R.Y.T.
www.myrehab.com

Integrative Yoga Therapy Training
www.iytyogatherapy.com
> A teacher training emphasizing a multi-systems approach to supporting students with health challenges.

Timothy McCall, M.D.
www.DrMcCall.com

Medical Editor for *Yoga Journal*. Writes online columns on yoga therapy.

Prime of Life Yoga
Larry Payne, Ph.D.
(800) 359-0171
www.samata.com
samatayoga@earthlink.net

Krishna Raman, M.D.
10, 12th Cross St. Indira Nagar
Chennai 600 020 India
91 44 2 490 0980
http://www.drkrishnaraman.com
mediyoga@vsnl.com

Rehab Yoga
Dalia Zwick, P.T.
www.rehabyoga.com
info@rehabyoga.com

Rehabyoga.com is an educational website designed to communicate the benefits of yoga for rehabilitating people with physical disability, their caregivers, and their therapists.

Sacred Space Health Center
Lori Newell M.A., C.P.T.
(508) 367-6311
www.sacredspacehealthcenter.com
email@sacredspacehealthcenter.com

Programs for people with chronic illness and post-rehabilitation needs.

Stone Center for Yoga & Health
Charlotte Chandler Stone (Hamsa)
(201) 833-5955
www.stoneyoga.com

   Charlotte is a Certified Structural Yoga Therapist with advanced training in working with those with osteoporosis and osteopenia.

Yoga and Breast Health Workshops
Joanna Colwell
www.ottercreekyoga.com
Joanna@ottercreekyoga.com

Yoga and Osteoporosis
Sara Meeks, Yoga and Physical Therapy
(888) 330-7272
www.sarameekspt.com
info@sarameekspt.com

Yoga for the Heart Training
Nischala Joy Devi
(415) 459-5336
www.abundantwellbeing.com
Nd@abundantwellbeing.com

   Nischala Joy Devi developed the pioneering yoga programs for Drs.
Dean Ornish and Michael Lerner. This course is for teachers and people
living with heart disease, cancer, and other debilitating diseases.

Yoga Therapy Center
Mukunda Stiles
(305) 442-7004
www.dynamicsystemsrehab.com
info@yogatherapycenter.org

Healthy Aging Websites

American Association of Retired* Persons
www.aarp.org

   *I vote for changing "Retired" to "Renewed," "Refreshed," "Re-energized,"
"Re-invented," or something like that!

Gray Panthers
(800) 280-5362 or (202) 737-6637
www.graypanthers.org
info@graypanthers.org

An advocacy organization promoting the rights of senior citizens, founded by the unforgettable Maggie Kuhn.

Living Over Aging
www.livingoveraging.com

Information on holistic gerontology.

National Institute on Aging
www.nia.nih.gov

Andrew Weil, M.D.
www.healthyaging.com

Offers the latest research on healthy aging.

Yoga Props

The companies listed here have excellent educational websites, catalogs, and instructional booklets that demonstrate the many uses of yoga props.

Sources for Yoga Wall Ropes

Gemini Track Wall Rope System
(805) 568-5309
www.goldentreeyoga.com
michael@goldentreeyoga.com

The Great Yoga Wall
(775) 781-0468
www.yogawall.com
info@yogawall.com

How to Use Wall Ropes

The booklet *Yoga Kurunta: An Exploration in the Use of Wall Ropes for the Practice of Yoga Asanas,* by Chris Saudek, is designed to be used under the guidance of an Iyengar yoga teacher. Available through Iyengar yoga websites, including www.customyogaprops.com.

Yoga Props
(888) 856-YOGA (9642)
www.yogaprops.net

A set of wall ropes comes with an instructional booklet: *The Yoga Props Wall Ropes Usage Guide* by E. Kay Eskenazi and Ruth Steiger.

Sources for Yoga Chairs and Other Props

Custom Yoga Props
(888) 870-2600 or (480) 642-8455
www.customyogaprops.com
customyogaprops@customyogaprops.com

A source for yoga chairs, wooden yoga props such as the horse, and other props.

Tools for Yoga
(888) 678-YOGA (9642)
www.toolsforyoga.net
staff@yogapropshop.com

Ropes, chairs, and more!

Miscellaneous Prop Sources

Bakti Bheka Yoga Supplies
(800) 366-4541
www.Bheka.com

Hugger-Mugger Yoga Products
(800) 473-4888
www.Huggermugger.com

YogaPro
(800) 488-8414
www.yogapro.com

Yoga Videos for Older Students and Their Teachers

Finding Felicity: The Life of Felicity Green
www.felicityoga.com

An inspiring video about senior teacher Felicity Green, one of my first teachers.

Lilias!
Lilias Folan
www.liliasyoga.com

Patricia Walden

Patricia Walden's videos can be found at www.yoga.com.

Yoga and the Gentle Art of Healing: A Journey of Recovery After Breast Cancer
Susan Rosen
(858) 481-3912
www.yogajoyofdelmar.com
susan@yogajoyofdelmar.com

Yoga at 92: The Bernard Spira Story
Shaw/Shapiro Productions
(310) 821-7844
www.senioryogis.org

Yoga for Blood Pressure
www.bsiyengar.com

Interactive multimedia CD. B. K. S. Iyengar describes a total of nineteen asanas with the specific sequence in which they need to be performed for low blood pressure and twenty-eight asanas for high blood pressure (hypertension). Gives simple explanations of what blood pressure is, what the common causes and abnormalities are, and more.

Yoga for Scoliosis with Elise Browning Miller
www.ebmyoga.com

This video/DVD by Elise B. Miller, scoliosis and back care expert, is the next best thing to taking a yoga workshop with her. The companion booklet alone is worth the cost.

Yoga for the Rest of Us
Peggy Cappy
www.peggycappy.com

Yoga for the Young at Heart with Susan Winter Ward
(800) 558-YOGA (9642)
www.yogaheart.com

Yoga Unveiled
www.yogaunveiled.com

DVD, produced by Gita Desai. *Yoga Unveiled* reveals how yoga began, tells the story of yoga's passage to the West, describes its numerous branches, recounts the fascinating biographies of the foremost yoga masters, and explores yoga's astonishing medical potential.

Yoga with Eric Small
www.yogaMS.com

Yoga for multiple sclerosis and other health challenges.

Note: *I receive many requests for videos on "chair yoga." These can be found on the Internet by searching for "chair yoga." Contact the organizations listed in this section for additional videos and audiotapes appropriate for older beginners.*

APPENDIX D

Bibliography

O ne of the perks of writing a book is that it gives you an excuse to read more books! Following is a list of the books, magazines, other publications, videos and additional sources of information consulted in the course of writing this book. I also include some additional titles that I think you will find useful. My reviews for many of these books are posted on www.amazon.com.

This bibliography is divided into five categories:

- Yoga

- Healthy Aging

- Conscious Dying and Death

- *Ahimsa* (Nonviolence)

- Journals, Magazines, Newsletters, and Other Publications

Yoga

Alberg, Maria. *The Yoga Workbook for Seniors*. Sandpoint, ID: Moon in the Pearl, 1993.

Austin, Miriam. *Cool Yoga Tricks*. New York: Ballantine/The Random House Publishing Group, 2003.

Bell, Lorna, R.N., and Eudora Seyfer. *Gentle Yoga for People with Arthritis, Stroke Damage, Multiple Sclerosis or People in Wheelchairs*. Berkley, CA: Celestial Arts, 1987.

Bender, Ruth. *Be Young and Flexible After 30, 40, 50, 60*. Avon, CT: Ruben Publishing, 1976.

Blaine, Sandy. *Yoga for Healthy Knees*. Berkeley, CA: Rodmell Press, 2005.

Brena, Steven. *Yoga & Medicine*. Baltimore, MD: Penguin Books, 1973.

Cappy, Peggy. *Yoga for All of Us*. New York: St. Martin's Press, 2006.

Christensen, Alice. *The Easy Does It Yoga Trainer's Guide*. Sarasota: FL: The American Yoga Association, 1995.

Christensen, Alice, and David Rankin. *Easy Does It Yoga for People Over 60*. Cleveland, OH: Saraswati Studio, 1975.

Claire, Thomas. *Yoga for Men: Postures for Healthy, Stress-Free Living*. Franklin Lakes, NJ: Career Press/New Age Books, 2004.

Clennell, Bobby. *Props and Ailments*. Self-published. bobbyclennell@aol.com. Can be ordered from www.yogaprops.net, www.iyengar-yoga.com, and other Iyengar yoga websites listed in Appendix C.

Cope, Stephen. *Yoga and the Quest for the True Self*. New York: Bantam Books, 1999.

Coulter, H. David. *Anatomy of Hatha Yoga: A Manual for Students, Teachers, and Practitioners*. Honesdale, PA: Body and Breath, Inc., 2001.

Criswell, Eleanor. *How Yoga Works: An Introduction to Somatic Yoga*. Novato, CA: Freeperson Press, 1987.

Desikachar, T. K. V. *The Heart of Yoga: Developing a Personal Practice*. Rochester, VT: Inner Traditions International, 1995.

Devi, Nischala Joy. *The Healing Path of Yoga: Time-Honored Wisdom and*

Scientifically Proven Methods that Alleviate Stress, Open Your Heart, and Enrich Your Life. New York: Three Rivers Press, 2000.

Dickman, Carol. "Bed Top Yoga" and "Chair Yoga." Yoga audiotapes for the blind and visually impaired, based on *Videos for Seniors*. www.yogaeze .com, carol@stretch.com.

Dworkis, Sam. "The Paradox of Younger Yoga Teachers," retrieved August 4, 2006, at www.extensionyoga.com/essays1.asp#Catch22.

———. *Extensions: The 20-Minute-a-Day, Yoga-Based Program to Relax, Release & Rejuvenate the Average Stressed-Out Over-35-Year-Old Body*. New York: Poseidon Press, 1994.

———. *Recovery Yoga: A Practical Guide for Chronically Ill, Injured, and Post-Operative People*. New York: Three Rivers Press, 1997.

Fishman, Loren Martin, and Eric Small. *Yoga and Multiple Sclerosis: A Journey to Health and Healing*. New York: Demos Medical Publishing, 2006.

Folan, Lilias. *Lilias! Yoga Gets Better with Age*. Emmaus, PA: Rodale Books, 2005.

Francina, Suza. *The New Yoga for People Over 50: A Comprehensive Guide for Midlife and Older Beginners*. Deerfield Beach, FL: Health Communications, Inc., 1997.

———. *Yoga and the Wisdom of Menopause: A Guide to Physical, Emotional and Spiritual Health at Midlife and Beyond*. Deerfield Beach, FL: Health Communications, Inc., 2003.

Frawley, David, and Sandra Summerfield Kozak. *Yoga for Your Type: An Ayurvedic Approach to Your Asana Practice*. Twin Lakes, WI: Lotus Press, 2001.

Heriza, Nirmala. *Dr. Yoga: Yoga for Health*. New York: Jeremy Tarcher/Penguin, 2004.

Holleman, Dona, and O. Sen-Gupta. *Dancing the Body of Light: The Future of Yoga*. The Netherlands: Pegasus Enterprises, 1999.

Iyengar, B. K. S. *Light on Yoga*. New York: Schocken, 1979.

———. *Light on Pranayama*. New York: Crossroad Publishing Co., 1981.

———. *Iyengar: His Life and Work*. Palo Alto, CA: Timeless Books, 1987.

———. *Tree of Yoga*. Boston: Shambhala, 1989.

———. *70 Glorious Years of Yogacharya B. K. S. Iyengar.* Bombay, India: Light on Yoga Research Trust, 1990.

———. *Light on the Yoga Sutras of Patanjali.* London: Harper Collins, 1993.

———. *Yoga: The Path to Holistic Health.* London: Dorling Kindersley Ltd., 2001.

———. *Light on Life: The Yoga Journey to Wholeness, Inner Peace, and Ultimate Freedom.* Emmaus, PA: Rodale Books, 2005.

Iyengar, Geeta S. *Yoga: A Gem for Women.* Spokane, WA: Timeless Books, 1990.

Iyengar, Prashant. *Alpha and Omega of Trikonasana.* Mumbai, India: Iyengar Yogashraya, 2004.

Joshua, Sholom. *The Hip Yoga Sutras.* Self-published. Ojai, CA. 2005.

Laird, Joan. *Ageless Exercise: A Gentle Approach for the Inactive or Physically Limited.* Grawn, MI: Angelwood Press. 1994.

Lasater, Judith Hanson, Ph.D., P.T. *Relax and Renew: Restful Yoga for Stressful Times.* Berkeley, CA: Rodmell Press, 1995.

———. *Living Your Yoga: Finding the Spiritual in Everyday Life.* Berkeley, CA: Rodmell Press, 2000.

———. *30 Essential Yoga Poses: For Beginning Students and Their Teachers.* Berkeley, CA: Rodmell Press, 2003.

———. *Yoga Abs: Moving from Your Core.* Berkeley, CA: Rodmell Press, 2005.

Lewis, Dennis. *Free Your Breath, Free Your Life: How Conscious Breathing Can Relieve Stress, Increase Vitality, and Help You Live More Fully.* Boston and London: Shambhala, 2004.

———. *The Tao of Natural Breathing: For Health, Well-Being, and Inner Growth.* Berkeley, CA: Rodmell Press, 2005.

Lowitz, Leza, and Reema Datta. *Sacred Sanskrit Words: For Yoga, Chant, and Meditation.* Berkeley, CA: Stone Bridge Press, 2005.

Maddern, Jan. *Yoga Builds Bones: Easy Gentle Stretches that Prevent Osteoporosis.* Boston, MA: Element Books, 2000.

McCall, Timothy, M.D. *Examining Your Doctor: A Patient's Guide to Avoiding Harmful Medical Care.* New York: Carol Publishing, 1996.

———. *Yoga as Medicine*. New York: Bantam Dell, 2007.

Mehta, Mira. *How to Use Yoga*. Berkeley, CA: Rodmell Press, 1998.

Mehta, Silvia, Mira Mehta and Shyam Mehta. *Yoga the Iyengar Way: The New Definitive Illustrated Guide*. New York: Knopf, 1990.

Miller, Elise Browning, and Carol Blackman. *Life Is a Stretch: Easy Yoga, Anytime, Anywhere*. St. Paul, MN: Llewellyn Publications, 2001.

———. *Yoga for Scoliosis*. Palo Alto, CA: Shanti Productions, 2003.

Moyer, Donald. *Yoga: Awakening the Inner Body*. Berkeley, CA: Rodmell Press, 2006.

Newborn, Barbara. *Return to Ithaca: A Young Woman's Triumph Over the Disabilities of a Severe Stroke*. Rockport, MA: Element Books, 1997.

Newell, Lori, M.A. *The Book of Exercise and Yoga for Those with Arthritis, Fibromyalgia and Related Conditions*. Harwichport, MA: Sacred Space Health Center, 2005.

Payne, Larry, Ph.D., and Richard Usatine, M.D. *Yoga Rx: A Step-by-Step Program to Promote Health, Wellness, and Healing for Common Ailments*. New York: Broadway Books, 2002.

Pegrum, Juliet. *Ageless Yoga: Gentle Workouts for Health & Fitness*. New York: Sterling Publishing, 2005.

Radha, Swami Sivananda. *Hatha Yoga: The Hidden Language*. Boston: Shambhala, 1987.

Raman, Krishna, M.D. *A Matter of Health: Integration of Yoga & Western Medicine for Prevention & Cure*. Madras, India: East West Books Pvt. Ltd., 1998.

———. and S. Suresh, M.D. *Yoga and Medical Science FAQ*. Madras, India: East West Books Pvt. Ltd., 2003.

Rosen, Richard. *Yoga for 50+: Modified Poses and Techniques for a Safe Practice*. Berkeley, CA: Ulysses Press, 2004.

Sanford, Matthew. *Waking: A Memoir of Transcendence*. Emmaus, PA: Rodale Press, 2006.

Saudek, Chris. *Yoga Kurunta: An Exploration in the Use of Wall Ropes for the Practice of Yoga Asanas*. La Crosse, WI: The Yoga Place, 2001.

Scaravelli, Vanda. *Awakening The Spine: The Stress-Free New Yoga that Works with the Body to Restore Health, Vitality and Energy.* San Francisco, CA: HarperCollins, 1991.

Schatz, Mary Pullig, M.D. *Back Care Basics: A Doctor's Gentle Yoga Program for Back and Neck Pain Relief.* Berkeley, CA: Rodmell Press, 1992.

Schiffmann, Erich. *Yoga: The Spirit and Practice of Moving into Stillness.* New York: Simon & Schuster, 1996.

Self, Philip. *Yogi Bare: Naked Truth from America's Leading Yoga Teachers.* Nashville, TN: Cypress Moon Press, 1998.

Shah, J. T., M.D. *Therapeutic Yoga.* Mumbai, India: Vakil, Feffer and Simons, Ltd., 1999.

Small, Eric. *See* Fishman, Loren Martin.

Sparrowe, Linda, and Walden, Patricia. *The Woman's Book of Yoga and Health: A Lifelong Guide to Wellness.* Boston, MA: Shambhala Publications, Inc., 2002.

———. *Yoga for Healthy Bones: A Woman's Guide.* Boston, MA: Shambhala Publications, Inc., 2004.

Stewart, Mary. *Yoga Over 50: The Way to Vitality, Health and Energy in the Prime of Life.* London: Little, Brown and Company, 1995.

Telang, Sulochana D., M.D. *Understanding Yoga Through Body Knowledge.* Pune, India: Padmagandha Prakashan, 1999.

Ward, Susan Winter. *Yoga for the Young at Heart: Gentle Stretching Exercises for Seniors.* Santa Barbara, CA: Capra Press, 1994.

Yogananda, Paramahansa. *Autobiography of a Yogi.* Los Angeles, CA: Self-Realization Fellowship, 1946.

Healthy Aging

Bianchi, Eugene C. *Aging as a Spiritual Journey.* New York: Crossroad Publishing Co., 1989.

Bolen, Jean Shinoda, M.D. *Crones Don't Whine: Concentrated Wisdom for Juicy Women.* Newburyport, MA: Conari Press, 2003.

Borysenko, Joan, Ph.D. *A Woman's Book of Life: The Biology, Psychology, and Spirituality of the Feminine Life Cycle.* New York: Penguin Putnam, Inc., 1996.

Brown, Susan E., Ph.D., and Russell Jaffe, M.D. *Better Bones, Better Body: Beyond Estrogen and Calcium*, 2nd ed. Lincolnwood, IL: Keats Publishing, 2000.

Chopra, Deepak. *Ageless Body, Timeless Mind: The Quantum Alternative to Growing Old*. New York: Harmony Books, 1993.

Crowley, Chris, and Henry S. Lodge, M.D. *Younger Next Year: A Guide to Living Like 50 Until You're 80 and Beyond*. New York: Workman Publishing, 2004.

Dychtwald, Ken, and Joe Flower. *Age Wave: The Challenges and Opportunities of an Aging America*. New York: Bantam Books, 1990.

Evans, William, Ph.D., Irwin H. Rosenberg, M.D., and Jacqueline Thompson. *Biomarkers: The 10 Keys to Prolonging Vitality*. New York: Simon & Schuster, 1991.

Hollis, James. *The Middle Passage: From Misery to Meaning in Midlife*. Toronto, Canada: Inner City Books, 1993.

Krucoff, Carol, and Mitchell Krucoff, M.D. *Healing Moves: How to Cure, Relieve, and Prevent Common Ailments with Exercise*. New York: Crown Publishing, 2000.

Ornish, Dean, M.D. *Dr. Dean Ornish's Program for Reversing Heart Disease*. New York: Random House, 1990.

Oz, Mehmet, M.D. *Healing from the Heart: A Leading Surgeon Combines Eastern and Western Traditions to Create the Medicine of the Future*. East Rutherford, NJ: Plume Books, 1999.

———. and Michael F. Roizen, M.D., *YOU: The Owner's Manual*. New York: HarperResource/HarperCollins Publishers, 2005.

Pelletier, Kenneth R. *Longevity: Fulfilling Our Biological Potential*. New York: Dell, 1981.

Pengrum, Juliet. *Ageless Yoga: Gentle Workouts for Health and Fitness*. New York: Sterling Publishing, 2006.

Price, Weston A., D.D.S. *Nutrition and Physical Degeneration*. New York: Harper & Brothers, 1939.

Ram Dass. *Still Here: Embracing Aging, Changing, and Dying*. New York: Berkeley Publishing Group/Penguin Putnam, Inc., 2000.

———. *Fierce Grace*, Zeitgeist Films, 2003.

Spilner, Maggie. *Prevention's Complete Book of Walking: Everything You Need to Know to Walk Your Way to Better Health*. Emmaus, PA: Rodale Books, 2000.

Wazen, Jack J., M.D. *Dizzy: What You Need to Know About Managing and Treating Balance Disorders*. New York: Fireside/Simon & Schuster, 2004.

Walker, Barbara G. *The Crone: Woman of Age, Wisdom, and Power*. San Francisco, CA: HarperCollins, 1985.

Weil, Andrew, M.D. *Healthy Aging: A Lifelong Guide to Your Physical and Spiritual Well-Being*. New York: Knopf, 2005.

Conscious Dying and Death

Ansley, Helen Green. *Life's Finishing School—What Now—What Next? A Ninety Year Old's View of Death and Dying a Good Death*. Sausalito, CA: Institute of Noetic Sciences, 1990.

Blackman, Sushila. *Graceful Exits: How Great Beings Die*. New York: Weatherhill, 1997.

Graber, Anya Foos. *Deathing: An Intelligent Alternative for the Final Moments of Life*, rev. ed., with a Preface by Ramamurti S. Mishra, M.D. York Beach, ME: Nicolas-Hays, 1992.

Krishnamurti, Jiddu. *On Living and Dying*. San Francisco, CA: Harper, 1992.

Kubler-Ross, Elisabeth. *Death: The Final Stage of Growth*. Englewood Cliffs, NJ: Prentice Hall, 1979.

Levine, Stephen. *Healing into Life and Death*. New York: Doubleday, 1987.

Nearing, Helen. *Loving and Leaving the Good Life*. Post Mills, VT: Chelsea Green Publishing, 1992.

Nuland, Sherwin B. *How We Die: Reflections on Life's Final Chapter*. New York: Vintage Books/Random House, 1993.

Ring, Kenneth. *Lessons from the Light*. Needham, MA: Moment Point Press, 2000.

———. *Life and Death*. New York: Coward, McCann & Geophegan, 1988.

Schacht, Maryann, M.S.W. *A Caregiver's Challenge: Living, Loving, Letting Go*. Lincoln, NE: Universe, 2004.

Sogyal Rinpoche. *The Tibetan Book of Living and Dying*. San Francisco: Harper, 1992.

Ahimsa (Nonviolence)

Eisnitz, Gail A. *Slaughterhouse: The Shocking Story of Greed, Neglect, and Inhumane Treatment Inside the U.S. Meat Industry*. Amherst, NY: Prometheus Books, 1997.

Gannon, Sharon. *Cats and Dogs Are People Too!* New York: Jivamukti Press, 1999.

The Humane Farming Organization, www.hfa.org.

People for the Ethical Treatment of Animals, www.Peta.org.

Journals, Magazines, Newsletters and Other Publications

Austin, Jacqueline, ed., *Light on Life Tour: Sri B. K. S. Iyengar Event Book*. San Francisco: Iyengar Yoga Association of Southern California, 2005.

Barret, Jenifer. "Heart to Heart," *Yoga Journal*, November/December 2003.

Bastille, Julie V., and Gill-Body, Kathleen M. "A Yoga-Based Exercise Program for People with Chronic Post Stroke Hemiparesis," *Physical Therapy*, vol. 84, no. 1, January 2004.

Bell, Baxter, M.D. "Yoga for Stroke Survivors," *Yoga Journal*, "Ask the Expert" article. Retrieved in 2006 at www.yogajournal.com/practice/967_1.cfm.

Bittorf, Rae. "Teaching Yoga to the Visually Impaired," *Yoga Rahasya*, vol. 9, no. 2, 2002.

Black, Kathryn. "Yoga Under the Microscope," *Yoga Journal*. Retrieved in 2006 at www.yogajournal.com/health/114_1.cfm.

Blank, Sally E., Ph.D., Kittel, Jacqueline, OTRL, R.Y.T., and Mel R. Haberman, Ph.D. "Active Practice of Iyengar Yoga as an Intervention for Breast Cancer Survivors," *International Journal of Yoga Therapy*, no. 15, 2005.

Carrico, Mara. "Yoga with a Chair," *Yoga Journal*, May/June 1986.

"Celebrating Community—Profiles: Felicity Green, Sandra Pleasants, Eleanor Williams, Elaine McGillicuddy, Francis McGillicuddy," *Yoga Samachar*, vol. 7, no. 1, Spring/Summer 2003.

Cogozzo, Linda. "Hatha After Hip Surgery," *Yoga Journal*, May/June 1985.

Cole, Roger, Ph.D. "Ask Our Expert: Practicing Safely with Bilateral Hip Replacements," *Yoga Journal*, retrieved 2006 at www.yogajournal.com/practice/596_1.cfm.

Desikachar, Kausthub, M.S., M.M.S. "The Yoga of Healing: Exploring Yoga's Holistic Model for Health and Well-Being: An Introduction," *International Journal of Yoga Therapy*, no. 15, 2005.

Dunn, Mary. "What Is the Best Way to Get Into and Out of Viparita Karani?" *Yoga Journal*, March/April 2004.

Faye, Laura. "Hard Work and Surrender," *LA Yoga, Ayurveda and Health Magazine*, vol. 4, no. 6, September/October 2005.

———. "Silver Age Yoga," *LA Yoga, Ayurveda and Health Magazine*, vol. 4, no. 6, September/October 2005.

Feuerstein, Georg, Ph.D. "Editorial: Whither Yoga Therapy?" *International Journal of Yoga Therapy*, no. 9, 1999.

———. "Yoga Therapy: Further Ruminations," *International Journal of Yoga Therapy*, no. 11, 2001.

Fishman, Loren Martin, M.D., and Eric Small. *Yoga and Multiple Sclerosis: A Journey to Health and Healing* (video). New York: Demos Medical Publishing, 2006.

Franklin, Ada-Reva, R.N., M.S.N., R.Y.T. "The Life Experiences of People with Multiple Sclerosis Who Practice Yoga: A Qualitative Case Study," *International Journal of Yoga Therapy*, no. 12, 2002.

French, Shirley Daventry. "Reflections," *Iyengar Yoga Centre of Victoria Newsletter*, May 2002, www.iyengaryogacentre.ca.

Garfinkel, Marian, Ph.D. "Carpal Tunnel Syndrome and Iyengar Yoga," *Yoga Rahasya*, vol. 10, no. 1, 2003.

Gilmore, Ruth, Ph.D. "The Effects of Yoga Asanas on Blood Pressure," *International Journal of Yoga Therapy*, no. 12, 2002.

Gudmestad, Julie. "Face Your Fears of Falling," *Yoga Journal*, July/August 2001.

———. "Break Out of Your Slump." *Yoga Journal*, November/December 2001.

———. "Bearing Up Under Pressure," *Yoga Journal*, May/June 2004.

Guthrie, Marisa. "Better with Age," *Yoga Journal*, May/June 2003.

Halis, Dale. "The Intelligence of Medical Yoga at Ramamani Iyengar Memorial Yoga Institute," *Yoga Therapy in Practice*, vol. 2, no. 1, February 2006.

Hansen, Patricia, M.A., R.Y.T., and Hansa Knox, B.S., L.M.T., R.Y.T. "The Gentle Loving Rehab of Yoga, with Ayurveda" *International Journal of Yoga Therapy*, no. 12, 2002.

Iyengar, B. K. S. "Yogacharya B. K. S. Iyengar Answers Questions on Aging," *Celebrating Longevity*, vol. 7, no. 1, Spring/Summer 2003.

Kelly, Alice Lesch. "Rest for the Weary," *Yoga Journal*, March/April 2001.

Kishiyama, Shirley, M.A., Jane Carlsen, B.A., Julie Lawrence, B.S., Eric Small, M.F.A., Daniel Zajdel, and Barry Oken, M.D. "Yoga as an Experimental Intervention for Cognition in Multiple Sclerosis," *International Journal of Yoga Therapy*, no. 12, 2002.

Kraftsow, Gary. "On Yoga Therapy," *Yoga International*, April/May 2002.

LePage, Joseph, M.A. "Creating Yoga Therapy Classes and Individual Sessions that Work," *International Journal of Yoga Therapy*, no. 12, 2002.

Lipson, Elaine. "Yoga Works!" *Yoga Journal*, Winter, 1999.

McCall, Timothy, M.D., "Count on Yoga: 38 Ways Yoga Keeps You Fit," *Yoga Journal*, January/February 2005.

McGonigal, Kelly. "Yoga Therapy in Practice," *International Journal of Yoga Therapy* (newsletter), Winter 2006.

Mehta, Rajvi, Ph.D. "Living Anatomy: Understanding the Hands," *Yoga Rahasya*, vol. 12, no. 4, 2005.

———. "Understanding Yoga Therapy," *International Journal of Yoga Therapy*, no. 12, 2002.

Miller, Amy Zone. "Living Proof: An Interview with Bernard Spira," *Yoga Vidya*, Spring/Summer 2005.

Miller, Tim, "How Yoga Can Prepare Us for Death," *Yoga Journal*. Retrieved in 2006 at www.yogajournal.com/practice/763_1.cfm.

Morrow, Shelly. "Joint Benefits," *Yoga Journal*, January/February 2002. (Article on yoga for arthritis featuring the work of Marian Garfinkel.)

Motiwala, Sam N. "Treating Chronic Ailments with Yoga: Constipation," *Yoga Rahasya*, vol. 9, no. 4, 2002.

Mureau, Heather L. "A Lesson in Teaching," *International Journal of Yoga Therapy*, no. 11, 2001.

Nelson, Steffie. "Yoga and Alzheimer's," *Yoga Journal*, March/April 2005.

Nett, Jaki. "Poses for Osteoporosis," *Yoga Journal*, "Ask the Expert," retrieved 2006 at www.yogajournal.com/practice/943_1.cfm.

Newborn, Barbara, M.A., R.Y.T. "Disability, Yoga and Transformation," *International Journal of Yoga Therapy*, no. 12, 2002.

Newell, Lori, M.A. "Combining Exercise with Yoga Postures, Breathing, and Meditation to Help Manage the Symptoms of Parkinson's Disease," *International Journal of Yoga Therapy*, no. 15, 2005.

Parry, Kay, and Julia Pedersen. "Seeing and Believing: A Photographic Glimpse and Point by Point Description of Guruji's Practice, February 2002," *Yoga Samachar*, vol. 7, no. 1, Spring/Summer 2003.

———. "Seeing and Believing: Guruji's Practice," *Yoga Samachar*, vol. 7, no. 2, Fall/Winter 2003.

———. "Seeing and Believing: Guruji's Practice." *Yoga Samachar*, vol. 8, no. 1, Spring/Summer 2004.

———. "Seeing and Believing: Guruji's Practice." *Yoga Samachar*, vol. 8, no. 2, Fall/Winter 2004.

Robin, Mel. "Reconciling Western Science and Iyengar Family Approach to Yoga Asana Practice," *Yoga Rahasya*, vol. 10, no. 3, 2003.

Robold, Libby, M.A., R.Y.T., and Patty Bauer, N.P. "Yoga and Hip Replacement Surgery," *International Journal of Yoga Therapy*, no. 15, 2005.

Saudek, Chris, and Francie Ricks. "Ageless Yoga," *Celebrating Longevity*, vol. 7, no. 1, Spring/Summer 2003.

Schatz, Mary, M.D. "Yoga Relief for Arthritis: A Pathologist and Yoga Teacher Offers Comprehensive Guidelines for Restoring and Maintaining Joint Health," *Yoga Journal*, May/June 1985.

————. "Exercises and Yoga Poses for Those at Risk for Osteoporotic Fractures," *Yoga Journal*, March/April 1988.

————. "You Can Have Healthy Bones! Preventing Osteoporosis with Exercise, Diet and Yoga," *Yoga Journal*, March/April 1988.

————. "Yoga and Aging," *Yoga Journal*, May/June 1990.

Serber, Ellen. "Carpal Tunnel Syndrome and Repetitive Stress: A Yogic Perspective," *International Journal of Yoga Therapy*, no. 9, 1999.

Stark, John. "Change Your Posture, Change Your Mood," *Yoga Journal*, July/August 2002.

Tawil, Rina. "Stabilizing Parkinson's Disease," *Yoga Rahasya*, vol. 10, no. 4, 2003.

Taylor, Matthew J., M.P.T., RYT. "Osteoporosis: An Opportunity to Serve," *International Journal of Yoga Therapy*, no. 15, 2005. Article on Yoga and Osteoporosis. Available online at www.iayt.org/site/publications/osteoporosis_taylor.pdf.

Tomasko, Felice M. "Yoga Goes to the Doctor?" *LA Yoga, Ayurveda and Health Magazine*, vol. 4, no. 2, March/April 2005.

Yoshikawa, Yoko. "Everybody Upside-Down," *Yoga Journal*, September/October 2000.

Zarthoshtimanesh, Zubin. "Modern Science Proving the Wisdom of the Sages," *Yoga Rahasya*, vol. 9, no. 2, 2002.

INDEX OF POSES

Author's Note: *This index does not list the more advanced postures demonstrated in this book. These are best learned under the guidance of a yoga teacher.*

Page numbers in *italics* indicate photographs.

INDEX

Page numbers in *italics* indicate photographs.

A

Adho Mukha Savasana
for arthritis, *149*, 150
  bone health and, 14
  daily practice and, 249–50, *250, 256,*
    256–58
  nervous system health and, 191
  as part of a typical class, 6, 9
  posture and, 184
  props for, *7, 37,* 43–44, *44,* 51, *52, 72,* 98
  wall ropes and, 92, *93, 94, 95, 96,*
    96–97, 104
Adho Mukha Vrkasana, 8, 135, 234
agility, 122
aging, xxiv–xxviii, 12, 20–25, 68
Ahimsa, 304–5, 306
alcohol, 118
alignment, 132, 311
Alper, Judith, 324
aluminum cookware, 118
Alzheimer's disease, 21, 339–40
Anatomy of Hatha Yoga, 192
Anusara yoga, 245
Apt, Marla, 66
Ardha Chandrasana, 6, *88, 89, 164,* 258, *265,*
  265–66
Ardha Halasana, 290, *297,* 297–99, *298*
arteriosclerosis, 19, 118
arthritis. *See also* joint health
  calcium supplements and, 118
  cautions/guidelines for, 144–46
  in the hips, knees, and hands, 146–51
  Jim Jacobs on, 154–58
  osteoarthritis, 115
  overview of, 138–40
  types of, 140
  yoga for, 140–46

arthroplasty, hip. *See* hip replacement
  surgery
artificial hips. *See* hip replacement surgery
asanas, 39–40
awareness, 146
Ayurveda, 30

B

baby boomers, aging of, xvii, xxv–xxvi
Backbender, 6, *7,* 57
Backbend Pose, 60, 190, 193–94, *194,*
  195–97
backbends
  Backbend Pose, 60, 190
  Bow Pose, *1*
  Bridge Pose, 170
  Camel Pose, *179, 235*
  Chest Opener for, *184, 185*
  endocrine health and, 122
  One-Legged King Pigeon Pose, *xxi*
  preparation for, *184, 185*
  props for, 6, *7,* 193–94, *194,* 195–97
  Supported Bridge Pose, *186,* 274, *276,*
    276–77
back problems. *See* spine health
Baddha Konasana
  advanced variation of, *217, 243*
  full pose, *325*
  hip replacement surgery and, *171*
  inversions and, 104
  meditation and, *327*
  as part of a typical class, 8
  props for, *56, 76, 77, 248, 267*
  Supported, *50*
balance, 24, 122, 145, 210
balancing poses
  benefits of, 24
  Tree Pose, *xxii,* 24, *71,* 170
benches, 42, 57

371

ABOUT THE AUTHOR

Suza Francina is the author of *The New Yoga for People Over 50: A Comprehensive Guide for Midlife and Older Beginners* (Health Communications, Inc., 1997) and *Yoga and the Wisdom of Menopause: A Guide to Physical, Emotional and Spiritual Health at Midlife and Beyond* (Health Communications, Inc., 2003). She is a graduate of the Iyengar Yoga Institute of San Francisco, a certified Iyengar yoga instructor, a member of the International Association of Yoga Therapists, and a Registered Yoga Teacher. She has over thirty years of experience in the fields of yoga and exercise therapy and is a consultant for research studies about yoga.

Suza's interest in yoga and health began many years ago when she worked as a home healthcare provider for elderly and convalescing people. This gave her the opportunity to observe firsthand the mental and physical changes that often occur in the later years of life.

Suza's first book, a completely different *Yoga for People Over 50*, was published in 1977. Suza's writing has appeared in numerous magazines, including *Yoga Journal, Prevention, AARP, Yoga for EveryBody, Yoga Vidya, Let's Live, Senior Life,* and numerous books, including *Women's Health Care: A Guide to Alternatives, The Holistic Health Handbook, American Yoga, The Arthritis Cure*

Fitness Solution, Living Your Yoga, The Rodale Book of Building Stronger Bones for Life, and *Prevention's Complete Book of Walking.* Her own books have been published in several languages, including German, Russian, and Portuguese.

Suza was born in 1949, in The Hague, Holland, and is of Dutch–Indonesian heritage. She lives in Ojai, California, a valley widely considered one of the most beautiful and sacred places on Earth. She is a former mayor of Ojai and a spokesperson for sustainable lifestyles.

Suza specializes in classes and workshops for people beginning yoga at midlife and older. She teaches yoga internationally to people of all ages in a wide variety of settings.

When not writing or teaching, Suza enjoys bicycling and practicing yoga outdoors, in nature. She is the mother of a grown son and daughter and feels fortunate to live where she is surrounded by trees, birds, crickets, rabbits, and frogs, with a family that includes several dogs, cats, and other sentient beings.

For information about Suza Francina's teaching schedule, visit www.suzafrancina.com.